CORE CONCEPTS *in* COLONOSCOPY

CORE CONCEPTS *in* COLONOSCOPY

EDITOR

Douglas G. Adler, MD, FACG, AGAF, FASGE
Associate Professor of Medicine
Director of Therapeutic Endoscopy
Gastroenterology and Hepatology
Huntsman Cancer Institute
University of Utah School of Medicine
Salt Lake City, Utah

CRC Press
Taylor & Francis Group
Boca Raton London New York

CRC Press is an imprint of the
Taylor & Francis Group, an **informa** business

First published 2014 by SLACK Incorporated

Published 2024 by CRC Press
2385 NW Executive Center Drive, Suite 320, Boca Raton FL 33431

and by CRC Press
4 Park Square, Milton Park, Abingdon, Oxon, OX14 4RN

CRC Press is an imprint of Taylor & Francis Group, LLC

Library of Congress Cataloging-in-Publication Data
Core concepts in colonoscopy / [edited by] Douglas Adler.
p. ; cm.
Includes bibliographical references and index.
(alk. paper)
I. Adler, Douglas G., 1969- editor of compilation.
[DNLM: 1. Colonoscopy. WI 520]
RC804.C64
616.3'407545--dc23

2014004464

ISBN: 9781617116148 (pbk)
ISBN: 9781003523307 (ebk)

DOI: 10.1201/9781003523307

Additional resources can be found at
https://www.routledge.com/9781617116148

Dedication

For my wife and children.

Contents

Acknowledgments

I would like to thank Carrie Kotlar and John Bond for their support and enthusiasm for this project at all phases of conception and development.

About the Editor

Douglas G. Adler, MD, FACG, AGAF, FASGE received his medical degree from Cornell University Medical College in New York, NY. He completed his residency in internal medicine at Beth Israel Deaconess Medical Center/Harvard Medical School, Boston, MA. Dr. Adler completed both a general gastrointestinal fellowship and a therapeutic endoscopy/ERCP fellowship at Mayo Clinic in Rochester, MN. He then returned to the Beth Israel Deaconess Medical Center for a fellowship in endoscopic ultrasound. Dr. Adler is currently an associate professor of Medicine and Director of Therapeutic Endoscopy at the University of Utah School of Medicine in Salt Lake City, UT. Working primarily at the University of Utah School of Medicine's Huntsman Cancer Institute, Dr. Adler focuses his clinical, educational, and research efforts on the diagnosis and management of patients with gastrointestinal cancers and complex gastrointestinal disease, with an emphasis on therapeutic endoscopy. He is the author of more than 200 scientific publications, articles, and book chapters and has published 3 other books about gastroenterology: *Curbside Consultation in GI Cancers for the Gastroenterologist: 49 Clinical Questions*, *Self-Expanding Stents in Gastrointestinal Endoscopy*, and *The Little GI Book: An Easily Digestible Guide to Understanding Gastroenterology*.

Contributing Authors

Todd H. Baron, MD (Chapter 8)
Professor of Medicine
Division of Gastroenterology & Hepatology
Director of Advanced Therapeutic Endoscopy
University of North Carolina
Chapel Hill, North Carolina

Kathryn R. Byrne, MD (Chapter 10)
Assistant Professor
Division of Gastroenterology and Hepatology
University of Utah School of Medicine
Salt Lake City, Utah

Jonathan Cohen, MD, FASGE, FACG (Chapter 12)
Division of Gastroenterology
New York University School of Medicine
New York, New York

Serag Dredar, MD (Chapter 6)
Sutter Medical
Yuba City, California

Tolga Erim, DO (Chapter 3)
Advanced Therapeutic Endoscopy
Digestive Disease Institute
Cleveland Clinic Florida
Weston, Florida

Norio Fukami, MD, AGAF, FACG, FASGE (Chapter 2)
Associate Professor of Medicine
Director of Endoscopic Ultrasound, Innovative Technology, and Endoscopic Oncology
Medical Co-Director of Digestive Health Center
Division of Gastroenterology and Hepatology
University of Colorado Anschutz Medical Campus
Denver, Colorado

Vivek Kaul, MD, FACG (Chapter 5)
Associate Professor of Medicine
Chief, Division of Gastroenterology and Hepatology
Center for Advanced Therapeutic Endoscopy
University of Rochester Medical Center/Strong Memorial Hospital
Rochester, New York

Gyanprakash Ketwaroo, MD (Chapter 3)
Division of Gastroenterology
Beth Israel Deaconess Medical Center
Boston, Massachusetts

C. Andrew Kistler, MD, PharmD (Chapter 6)
Jefferson University School of Medicine
Philadelphia, Pennsylvania

Shivangi Kothari, MD (Chapter 5)
Assistant Professor of Medicine
Division of Gastroenterology and Hepatology
Center for Advanced Therapeutic Endoscopy
University of Rochester Medical Center
Rochester, New York

Linda S. Lee, MD (Chapter 11)
Director, Women's Health in GI and Endoscopic Education
Division of Gastroenterology, Hepatology and Endoscopy
Brigham and Women's Hospital
Assistant Professor of Medicine
Harvard Medical School
Boston, Massachusetts

John G. Lieb II, MD (Chapter 1)
Assistant Professor of Clinical Medicine
University of Pennsylvania
Director of Interventional Endoscopy,
Philadelphia Veterans Affairs Medical Center
Philadelphia, Pennsylvania

Douglas Pleskow, MD, AGAF, FASGE (Chapter 3)
Associate Clinical Professor of Medicine
Harvard Medical School
Co-Director of Endoscopy
Beth Israel Deaconess Medical Center
Boston, Massachusetts

Waqar Qureshi, MD, FRCP (Chapter 4)
Baylor University College of Medicine
Houston, Texas

John R. Saltzman, MD, FACP, FACG, FASGE (Chapter 11)
Director of Endoscopy
Brigham and Women's Hospital
Associate Professor of Medicine
Harvard Medical School
Gastroenterology Division
Boston, Massachusetts

Robert E. Sedlack, MD, MHPE (Chapter 9)
Associate Professor of Medicine
Mayo Clinic
Rochester, Minnesota

Ali Siddiqui, MD (Chapter 6)
Jefferson University School of Medicine
Philadelphia, Pennsylvania

Anna Strongin, MD (Chapter 6)
Thomas Jefferson University Hospital
Philadelphia, Pennsylvania

Shou-Jiang Tang, MD (Chapter 6)
Director of Therapeutic Endoscopy & Endoscopic Research
Associate Professor in Medicine
Division of Digestive Diseases
University of Mississippi Medical Center
Jackson, Mississippi

Jeffrey L. Tokar, MD (Chapter 7)
Fox Chase Cancer Center/Temple University Health System
Division of Gastroenterology
Philadelphia, Pennsylvania

Melissa A. Verrengia, MD (Chapter 7)
Temple University Health System
Division of Gastroenterology
Philadelphia, Pennsylvania

Nicolas Villa, MD (Chapter 4)
Baylor University College of Medicine
Houston, Texas

Louis M. Wong Kee Song, MD (Chapter 8)
Division of Gastroenterology and Hepatology
Mayo Clinic
Rochester, Minnesota

PREFACE

Colonoscopy is humbling. Even the most skilled and experienced endoscopists among us have found it difficult to navigate the sigmoid colon, reduce a loop, or reach the cecum. Expert endoscopists will miss polyps and even cancers; everyone, eventually, will cause a colonic perforation.

In the face of such realities, endoscopists must fall back on the core concepts of colonoscopy time and again to guide us through these difficulties to accomplish our goals in the course of caring for our patients. I know from my own experience that it was reading and thinking about the fundamentals of colonoscopy, combined with ongoing active colonoscopy practice, that allowed my skills to grow exponentially over time. As an experienced therapeutic endoscopist who has trained a large number of fellows to perform all manner of colonoscopy for many years, I have seen that mastery of these core concepts is the number one factor that allows clinical and procedural success on a regular basis.

In that light, this book aims to address and convey these core concepts of colonoscopy: from the structure and function of the colonoscope itself, to insertion techniques, loop formation and reduction, polypectomy techniques for any situation, the avoidance and management of perforations and other adverse events, and advanced techniques including (but not limited to) endoscopic mucosal resection and colonic stenting. Each chapter is illustrated lavishly with key images to accentuate and illustrate its main findings. The chapters also are accompanied by videos to illustrate basic and advanced colonoscopic techniques from many leading experts. I have made every effort to include a plethora of tips, tricks, and accumulated points of wisdom in each chapter to help the reader learn all facets of colonoscopy.

This book is aimed at a wide audience, including novice endoscopists, advanced trainees, and clinicians at all levels of practice. This volume will be particularly helpful to those currently in training or those who have completed training recently, but even senior clinicians will find a wealth of valuable material between these covers, especially given the many new technologies and techniques that have arisen in the past few years.

I hope the readers of this volume take full advantage of the wisdom from its authors and apply that knowledge in their daily colonoscopy practice for many years to come.

Douglas G. Adler, MD, FACG, AGAF, FASGE
Salt Lake City, Utah

1

The Structure and Function of the Modern Colonoscope

John G. Lieb II, MD

The foundation of the modern colonoscope dates back to the 1800s, when a man-made light source was attached to devices used to peer inside the human body that had been in use since the days of the Roman Empire. It was not until the 1950s, with the discovery of a practical means of bundling fiberoptic fibers together to generate an image, that a workable flexible colonoscope was developed.[1] Furthermore, it was not until 1969 that the entire human colon was viewed with a practical, workable, modern flexible colonoscope.[2]

Since then, a bewildering array of colonoscopes has emerged from various manufacturers from all corners of the world, each with a slightly different construction that can be dizzying to the novice endoscopist, although in practice the operation of these devices is remarkably similar. This chapter reviews the structure and function of the modern flexible colonoscope with an emphasis on outlining the similarities and differences among the most commonly encountered models.

Many of us can recall our first encounter with a colonoscope, likely during medical school, when a gastroenterology fellow may have taken us aside during a rare quiet moment in the endoscopy suite and let us hold the magical black camera. I remember noting with some satisfaction how air could be bubbled through the colonoscope when the tip was held under water and how to deflect the tip itself in several directions. Although that initial contact may have been an early emotional high point, I think my relationship with the colonoscope hit an all-time low within the first few days of my own gastroenterology fellowship when I learned that I had assembled the colonoscope improperly (in the intensive care unit and in the middle of the night) before attempting an emergency procedure. After that inauspicious start, I made it a point to understand the setup and operation of the colonoscope inside and out. Today I find satisfaction in teaching new (and sometimes

Adler DG, ed.
Core Concepts in Colonoscopy (pp 1-11).

experienced) technicians, nurses, gastrointestinal fellows, and attending physicians some insider features of colonoscope structure and function that allow the user to get some extra degree of utility from the device.

This chapter aims to demystify the structure and function of the flexible colonoscope and thereby ease trainee transitions to the endoscopy suite. Despite the fact that gastroenterologists use these devices on a daily basis, even senior operators may not fully understand the internal makeup of their colonoscopies, further emphasizing that a complete understanding of these devices is critically important.[3]

Common Structure and Function

All modern colonoscopes are divided into 5 main subassemblies, each with a specific purpose and connected in sequence. These are the control head, insertion tube, endoscope tip, umbilical cord, and, finally, an endoscope plug that connects the colonoscope itself to the light source/image processor. None of these subassemblies is designed to be removable in the endoscopy suite—all are attached to one another.

Control Head

The control head is the mechanical interface between the colonoscope and left hand of the operator. It contains the biopsy channel insertion orifice, the colonoscope control wheels, buttons to control picture quality and capture images, and the air/water and suction valves buttons (Figure 1-1). The biopsy channel, which can also be thought of as a second access point to the suction channel, is located just below the hand grip on the control head.

The biopsy channel, also referred to as the *working channel*, is the part of the colonoscope that allows passage of endoscopic devices (such as snares, needles, nets, forceps, and clips) through the entire length of the colonoscope and into the bowel lumen. The size of the channel dictates which devices can be passed; some colonoscopes (such as pediatric versions) have a somewhat narrow working channel, whereas other devices have a *therapeutic channel*, which allows passage of larger devices such as colonic stents. Forceful attempts at passing devices that are too large for the working channel can result in damage to both these devices and the colonoscope itself. In rare cases, the working channel can become perforated, rendering the colonoscope unsafe for further use until repaired.

The control head also includes the control wheels that allow the endoscopist to deflect the tip of the colonoscope on at least 2 axes (Figure 1-2). On forward-viewing endoscopes such as colonoscopes, the larger wheel (sometimes referred to as the *big wheel* or *vertical ratchet*) allows the tip of the endoscope to be moved in the vertical plane, creating up and down deflection. The smaller control wheel (also referred to as the *little wheel* or the *lateral ratchet*) allows left and right endoscope tip deflection. These wheels typically each have a locking function; this allows the operator to secure either or both wheels in position if extra stability is required during operation. The large wheel lock is located medially to the large wheel itself, whereas the little wheel lock is located laterally to the little wheel itself. It should be observed that the wheel locks do not freeze the top of the endoscope—the locks can be overcome by intentional movement of the control wheels against resistance. In general, the wheel locks are not commonly used during insertion of the endoscope and are of greatest value when performing maneuvers that require minimal to no endoscope

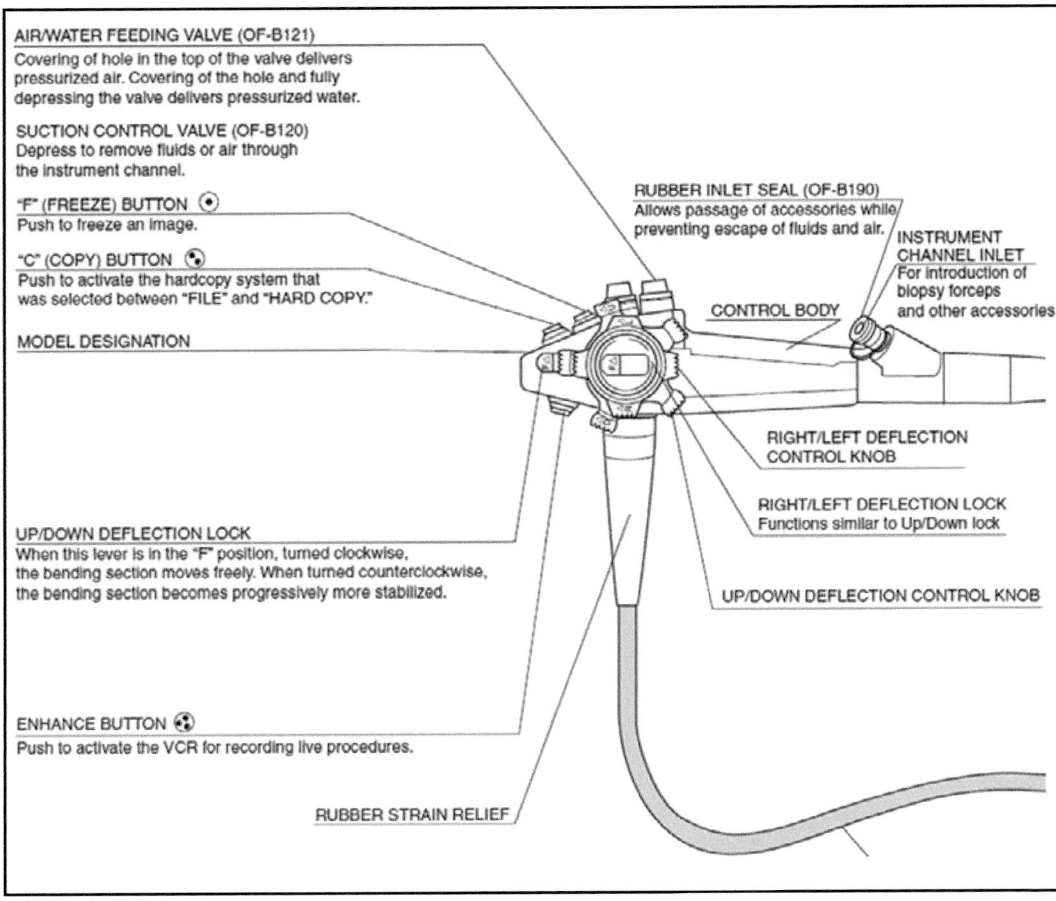

Figure 1-1. Schematic of colonoscope control head. (Reprinted with permission of Pentax Medical.)

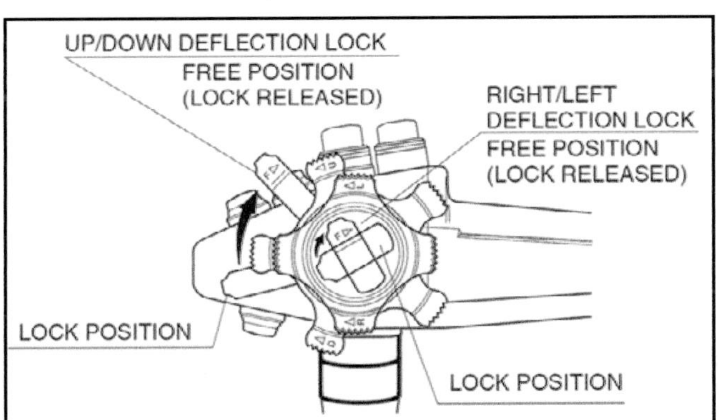

Figure 1-2. Schematic view of control wheels and wheel locks. (Reprinted with permission of Pentax Medical.)

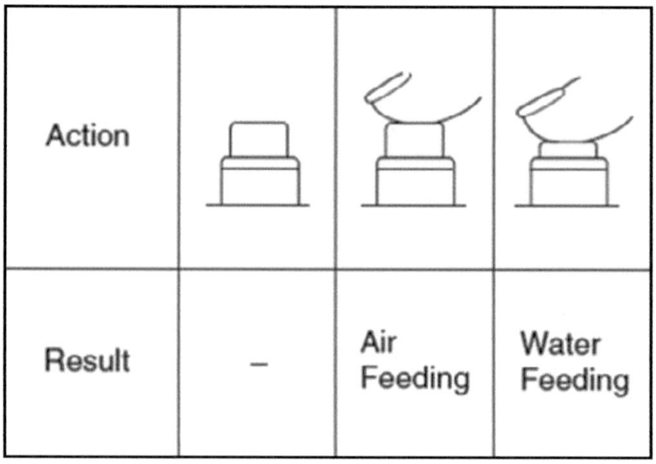

Figure 1-3. Schematic view of air/water valve operation. (Reprinted with permission of Pentax Medical.)

tip motion, such as during polypectomy or when attempting to stop bleeding. Rarely, the wheel locks can become activated inadvertently during normal use, and any unexpected sensation of resistance to control wheel movement should prompt the user to make sure the wheel locks are not activated.

The top of the control head also houses several buttons that allow the operator to freeze the current image on the screen for detailed viewing or capture the image for inclusion in the procedure report. Some endoscope models have buttons that allow image enhancements, such as image magnification or the activation of narrow band imaging.

The control head also contains 2 removable buttons into which mechanical valves are incorporated. One of these valves allows air and/or water to be suctioned, whereas the other allows air insufflation. The suction valve is activated when it is depressed. The air/water valve allows the operator to instill air into the patient and clean the endoscope's optical lens. Air is passed through the channel by covering the opening of the valve while the endoscope's optical lens is cleaned by water when depressing the air valve (Figure 1-3). In all modern colonoscopes, the suction valve is located above the air/water valve. The suction valve is operated by the index finger, and the air/water valve is operated by the middle finger. The air/water valve in particular tends to have sensitive o-rings, which can leak over time and become dysfunctional, and the suction valve can become clogged by stool particles during operation. Faulty valves can be replaced during a colonoscopy without disruption of the procedure. During the brief interval when the valves are being replaced, especially the air/water valve, the endoscope may leak or spray water on the operator, patient, or assistants. During a colonoscopy, the operator uses the index and middle fingers to depress the suction button and the air/water buttons, respectively (Figure 1-4).

Insertion Tube

The insertion tube is the long flexible portion of the colonoscope. The insertion tube houses the air/water/suction channels, the mechanical cables that connect the colonoscope tip to the control wheels, and most of the optical components. The insertion tube originates just below the control head, and the point where these 2 parts of the colonoscope meet can be damaged by severe angulation of this joint.

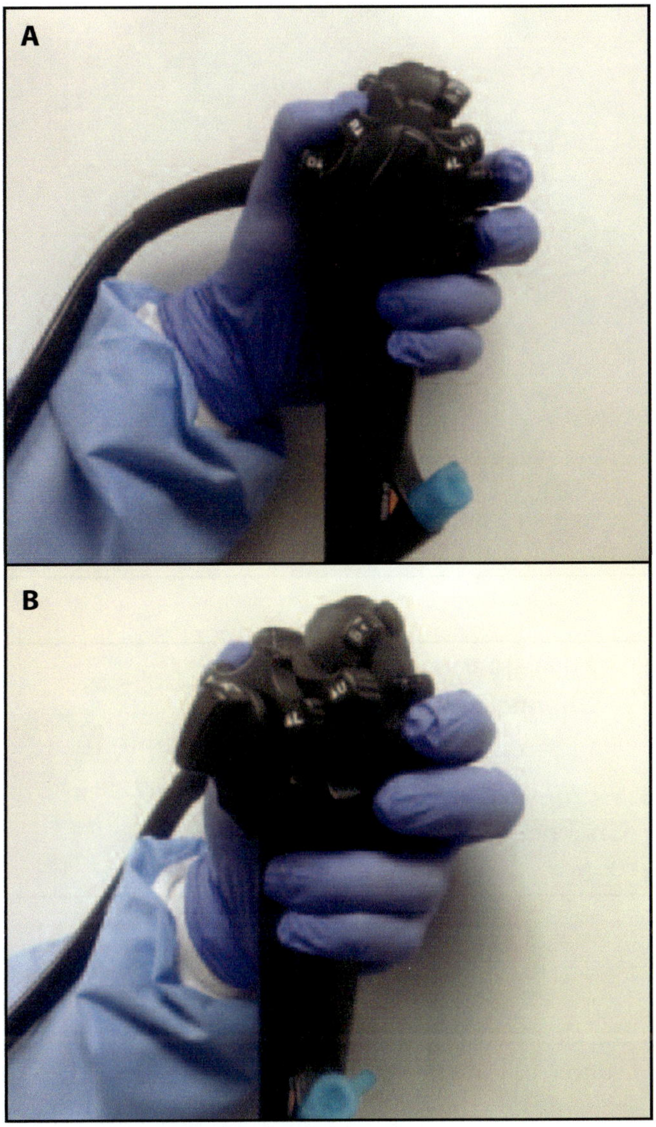

Figure 1-4. Proper hand positioning for holding a colonoscope control head. (A) Side view. (B) Oblique view emphasizing finger positions over the suction and air/water valve buttons. (Reprinted with permission of Douglas G. Adler, MD, FACG, AGAF, FASGE.)

Colonoscopes manufactured by Olympus America, Inc, also include a rotatable control wheel at the base of the control head just above the origin of the insertion tube that allows the operator to adjust the stiffness of the insertion tube. Such devices are known as variable-stiffness colonoscopes (Figure 1-5). This wheel can be used to tighten or loosen the control cables in the colonoscope during operation and is often used to help navigate tight turns or to minimize the formation of loops during a colonoscopy. In practice, variable-stiffness colonoscopes allow the operator to stiffen the insertion tube during advancement. The variable stiffness wheel generally is relaxed during colonoscopic withdrawal to maximize visualization and minimize trauma to the colonic mucosa. The insertion tube on adult colonoscopes tends to have a bit more intrinsic stiffness than that on pediatric colonoscopes, and stiffness can vary slightly from brand to brand and even among endoscopes from the same manufacturer. Older colonoscopes also may lose some degree of insertion tube stiffness over time from use, cable laxity, and other factors.

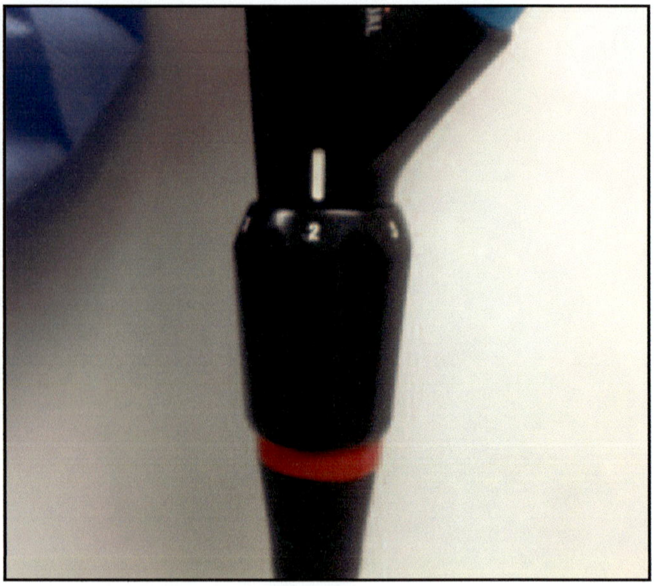

Figure 1-5. Close-up view of a base of the insertion tube on a variable-stiffness colonoscope. Note the rotatable cuff to adjust insertion tube shaft stiffness. (Reprinted with permission of Douglas G. Adler, MD, FACG, AGAF, FASGE.)

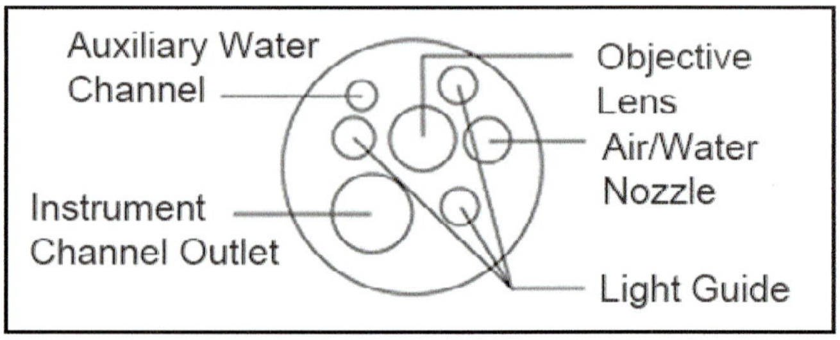

Figure 1-6. Schematic view of a colonoscope tip. (Reprinted with permission of Pentax Medical.)

Endoscope Tip

At the end of the colonoscope is the flexible tip, which can be deflected in 2 dimensions. From this, light from the light source illuminates the inside of the patient. Modern colonoscopes have 2 or 3 light channels in the endoscope tip that are fed by light fiber bundles connected to the light bulb in the light source/processor. The endoscope tip also contains the orifice of the working channel, water channel, optical lens, and lens-cleaning apparatus. The suction channel typically occupies the largest amount of space on the endoscope (Figure 1-6).

The endoscope tip is highly flexible and can bend fully back upon itself so the operator can perform the maneuver known as *retroflexion*, which is commonly employed in the rectum so the operator can visualize the most distal portion of the rectal lumen (Figure 1-7). Retroflexion can also be employed in the right colon to enhance polyp detection. Colonoscopes may have a lesser degree of tip deflection compared with upper endoscopes, but all of these devices can retroflex safely in clinical practice.

An important consideration is the field of view offered by the camera at the end of the endoscope tip. Commonly available colonoscopes provide 140 to 170 degrees of view (Figure 1-8). It is unclear whether a greater field of view allows the operator to identify more polyps, although devices with a greater field of view may reduce insertion times during colonoscopy.[4] Wide-view colonoscopes are an area of great interest, with single-lens

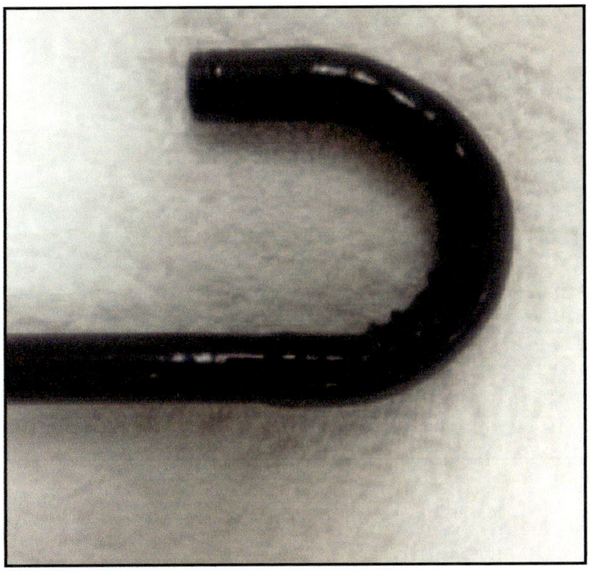

Figure 1-7. Close-up view of a colonoscope tip during retroflexion. (Reprinted with permission of Douglas G. Adler, MD, FACG, AGAF, FASGE.)

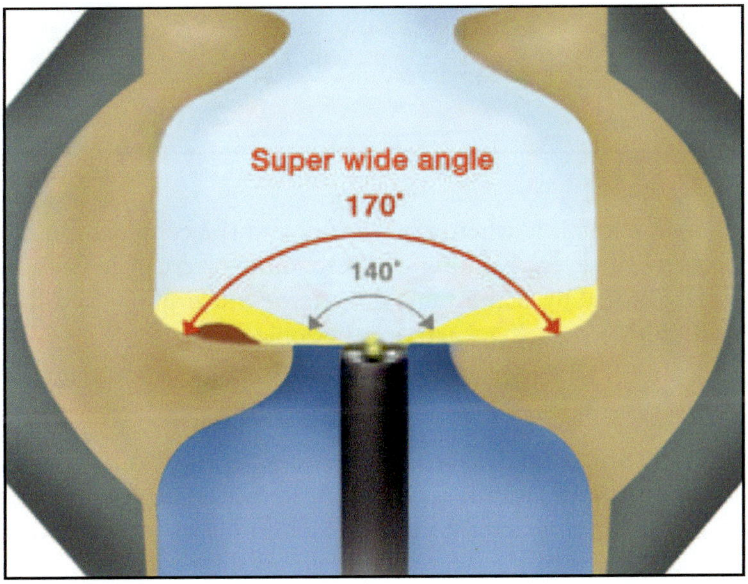

Figure 1-8. Diagram showing the difference between a 140- and 170-degree field of view. (Reprinted with permission of Olympus America, Inc.)

instruments offering a 230-degree view and multi-lens instruments offering up to a 330-degree view (Fuse Colonoscope; EndoChoice) (Figure 1-9). Multi-lens instruments require multiple monitors and are just now becoming available.[5]

Umbilical Cord

The umbilical cord attaches to the control head at a right angle and lies across the dorsal part of the operator's left hand, between the thumb and forefinger (Figures 1-10 and 1-11). The umbilical cord connects the colonoscope to the plug that allows it to join with the light source/processor. The attachment points of the umbilical cord with the control

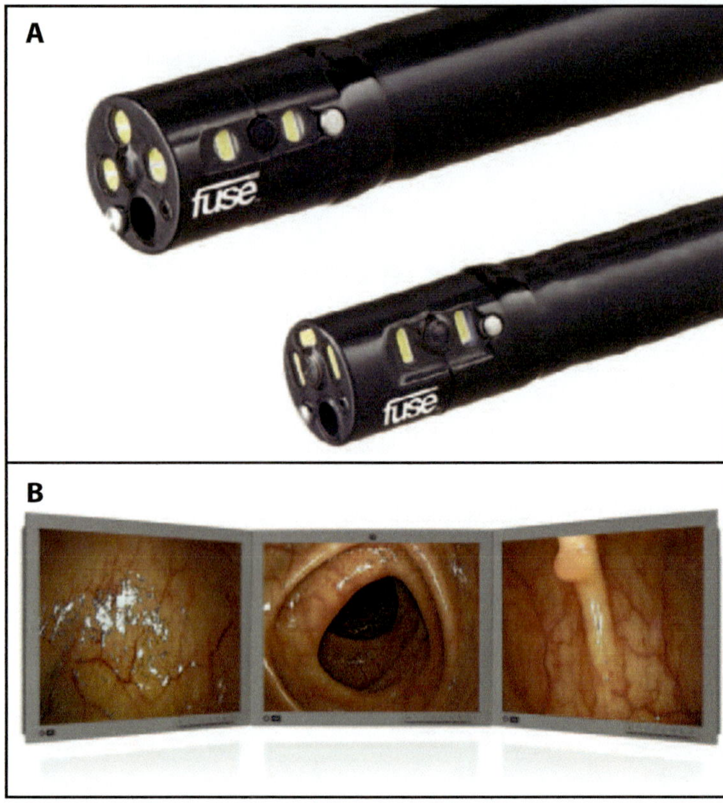

Figure 1-9. (A) Fuse colonoscope and upper endoscope tips, showing lenses and light sources at the sides and tips of the endoscopes. (B) Endoscopic view through the Fuse colonoscope, with 3 monitors giving a 330-degree view of the colon. (Reprinted with permission of EndoChoice, Inc.)

head and the plug are both vulnerable points where fiber optics and the colonoscope can be damaged. Damage can occur with severe bending of these joints or crush injuries to the umbilical cord itself (typically caused by slamming a door across the umbilical cord or running over the umbilical cord with a stretcher, cart, or other object).

Endoscope Plug

The endoscope plug connects the umbilical cord to the light source/processor. The plug also serves as the attachment point for air, water, and suction hoses to the colonoscope (Figure 1-12). Standard suction tubing connected to a wall suction outlet is attached to the plug's suction port, usually on the side of the plug. Water, supplied by a separate water bottle, is attached to the side of the colonoscope plug with 2 prongs that connect to a water irrigation tube. Some colonoscopes have a separate attachment point for a water lavage system; such a system allows the operator to instill a large volume of water into the colon quickly with a separate water pump. These lavage systems are separate from the water bottle used for lens cleaning.

Modern colonoscope systems contain a valve that minimizes or eliminates backflow of enteric contents into the water bottle and irrigation tubing. Improper use of this device (or lack of use of this device altogether) is thought to be responsible for several highly publicized cases of patient contamination and infection by enteric contents.[6]

The connection between the colonoscope and light source and optical fibers is usually attached to the plug via a large round connector piece that twists into position. Caution should be used when connecting the colonoscope to the light source and optics; the

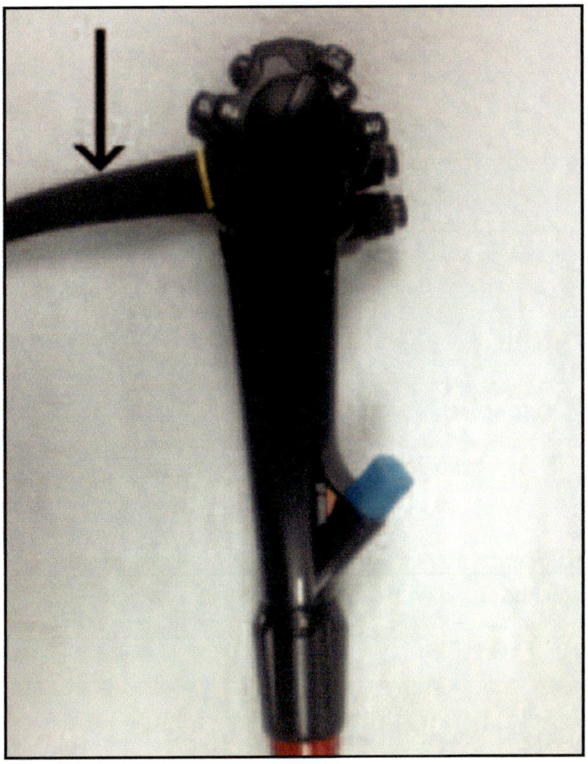

Figure 1-10. Umbilical cord (arrow) inserting into the control head of a colonoscope at a right angle. (Reprinted with permission of Douglas G. Adler, MD, FACG, AGAF, FASGE.)

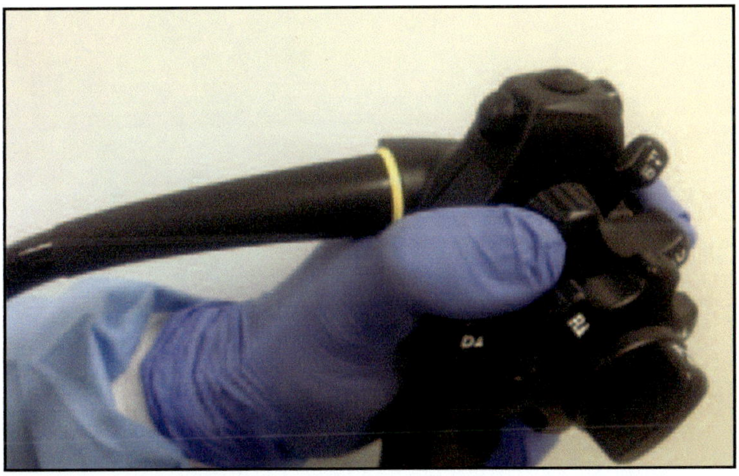

Figure 1-11. Umbilical cord resting between the thumb and index finger of the left hand. (Reprinted with permission of Douglas G. Adler, MD, FACG, AGAF, FASGE.)

delicate electrical connections can be bent and damaged with improper or forceful plug manipulation. This connector should not be submersed in liquid because it provides the electrical conductivity for the entire colonoscope. Accidental submersion of the plug can lead to irreversible colonoscope damage.

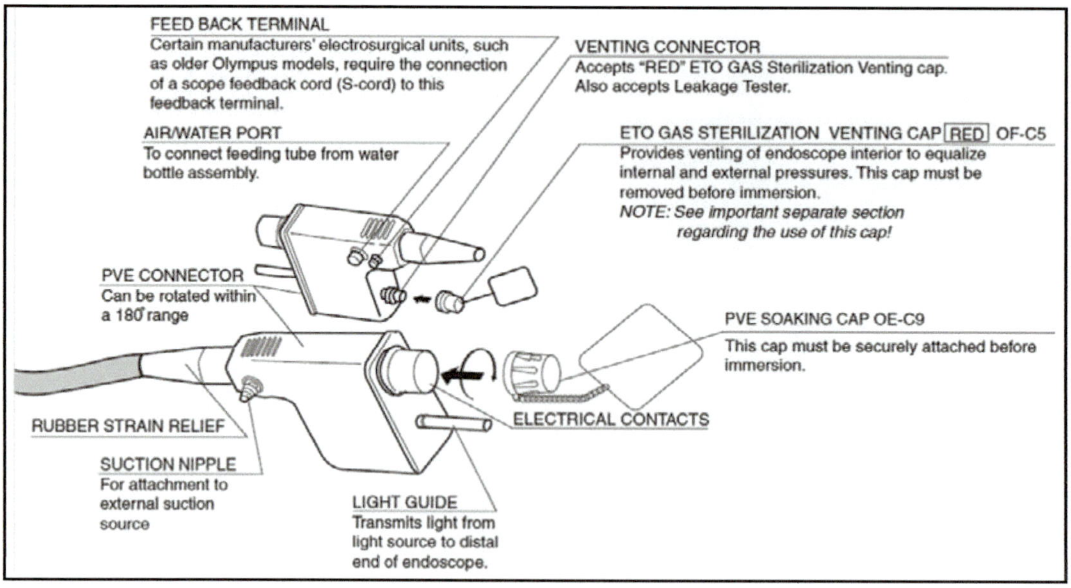

Figure 1-12. Schematic view of a colonoscope plug. (Reprinted with permission of Pentax Medical.)

Table 1-1. Differences Between Commonly Used Models

COLONOSCOPE TYPE	FUJINON	PENTAX	OLYMPUS
Colonoscope working length, mm	1330 to 1690	1700	1680
Colonoscope width, mm	12.8	14.6	13.9
Field of view, degrees	140	140	170
Number of lights on tip	2	2	3
Working channel diameter, mm	3.8	3.7	3.8

Key Differences Among Colonoscopes

Generally speaking, there are only subtle differences between commercially available colonoscopes (Table 1-1). Different manufacturers provide slightly different button, wheel, and valve shapes, but all are similar enough that knowledge of the operation of one endoscope allows competent operation of all other available colonoscopes. Different manufacturers may provide proprietary image enhancement features and slightly different button locations and image capture features. The variable-stiffness feature discussed previously is available only on Olympus colonoscopes.

Conclusion

Modern colonoscopes are significantly complex devices that allow physicians to perform a tremendous range of diagnostic and therapeutic maneuvers. The modern colonoscope is an amalgamation of several key mechanical parts that are merged into a single device. A thorough understanding of all of these parts is critical for procedural and technical success.

References

1. Edmonson JM. History of the instruments for gastrointestinal endoscopy. *Gastrointest Endosc.* 1991;37(suppl 2):S27-S56.
2. Wolff WI. Colonoscopy: history and development. *Am J Gastroenterol.* 1989;84(9):1017-1025.
3. Ott BJ, Nelson B. The structure and function of colonoscope channels: the inside story. *Gastroenterol Nurs.* 1998;21(2):48-51.
4. Deenadayalu VP, Chadalawada V, Rex DK. 170 degrees wide-angle colonoscope: effect on efficiency and miss rates. *Am J Gastroenterol.* 2004;99(11):2138-2142.
5. Uraoka T, Tanaka S, Matsumoto T, et al. A novel extra-wide-angle–view colonoscope: a simulated pilot study using anatomic colorectal models. *Gastrointest Endosc.* 2013;77(3):480-483.
6. Federal Health Matters series. VA report says endoscope reprocessing issues continue. *Federal Practitioner.* 2009;26(7):32-33.

2

Enhanced Imaging Techniques
What They Can and Cannot Do and When to Use Them

Norio Fukami, MD, AGAF, FACG, FASGE

Enhanced imaging techniques have been used for many years to assist in visual endoscopic inspection. Since it was first described by Tada et al[1] in 1977, dye spraying onto the mucosa has been the mainstay of these enhancements. Recently, more modern modalities to enhance mucosal details have emerged, and clinical data showing the efficacy of these modalities are beginning to accumulate.

Overview of Available Technologies

Chromoendoscopy is an enhancement method that traditionally has been accomplished by spraying a special dye onto the surface of the colonic mucosa. Two distinct mechanisms are used in the colon to enhance imaging: the absorptive staining method and the contrast method.

The staining method uses dye absorbed by the cells (ie, methylene blue and crystal violet), and the contrast method uses dye that goes into surface crevices to enhance groove pattern and color (for instance, the redness of blood vessels can be made more prominent).[2] In the colon, crystal violet is used to enhance visualization of magnification endoscopy to clarify the Kudo type V pit pattern and the invasive pattern, which are frequently used to determine whether there is deeper tumor invasion into the submucosa (Figures 2-1 to 2-3 and Table 2-1).[3-5]

Dye use has been reported mostly in Asia, and it is rarely used in the United States or Europe. The obstacles to using this technique include the lack of training for its effective use and its prolonged procedure time and associated costs. The use of dye requires additional medications (dye substance) and equipment (spray catheter and/or a syringe).

Adler DG, ed.
Core Concepts in Colonoscopy (pp 13-26).

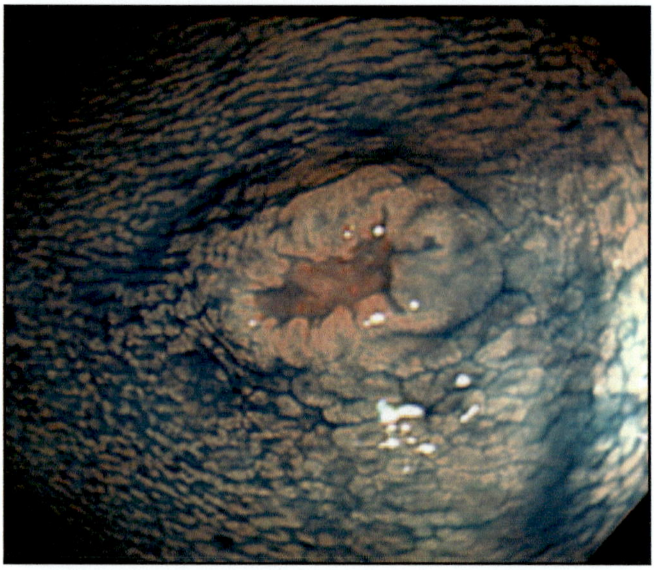

Figure 2-1. Depressed-type polyp in the colon is viewed after indigo carmine dye spray. Dye spray emphasizes depressed areas.

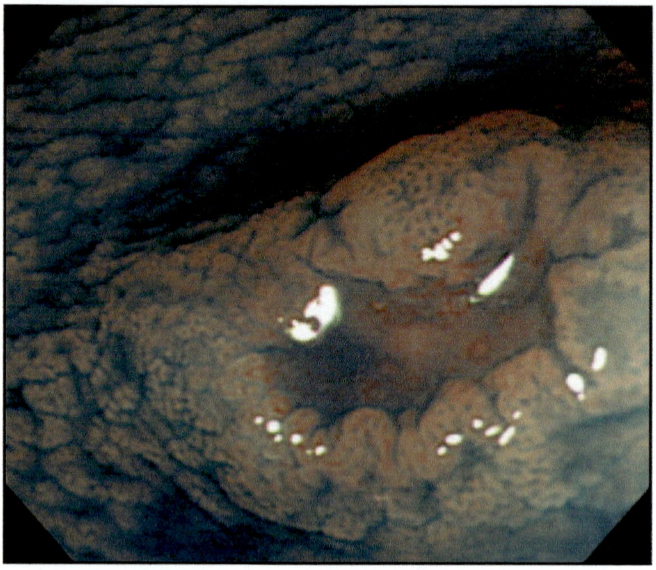

Figure 2-2. Closer view of the depressed-type polyp in Figure 2-1. The depressed area shows an ill-defined pit pattern.

However, chromoendoscopy has been shown to improve dysplasia detection in patients with inflammatory bowel disease (IBD), and thus its use is recommended in screening for dysplasia in patients with IBD (Figures 2-4 to 2-6).[6]

A newer technology, known as *narrow band imaging* (NBI), has emerged for visualization, which enhances blood vessels.[7] This method narrows the delivered light spectrum to only 2 major wavelengths, 440 to 460 nm (blue) and 540 to 560 nm (green), at which the light is absorbed by hemoglobin (thus darkening the blood vessels). Because blood vessels follow the villous and glandular structures, creating mucosal microvasculature, NBI also enhances the surface pattern of the mucosa (Figures 2-7 and 2-8).

Other types of imaging enhancement have been made commercially available. However, they use postimaging processing techniques that are different from NBI; that is,

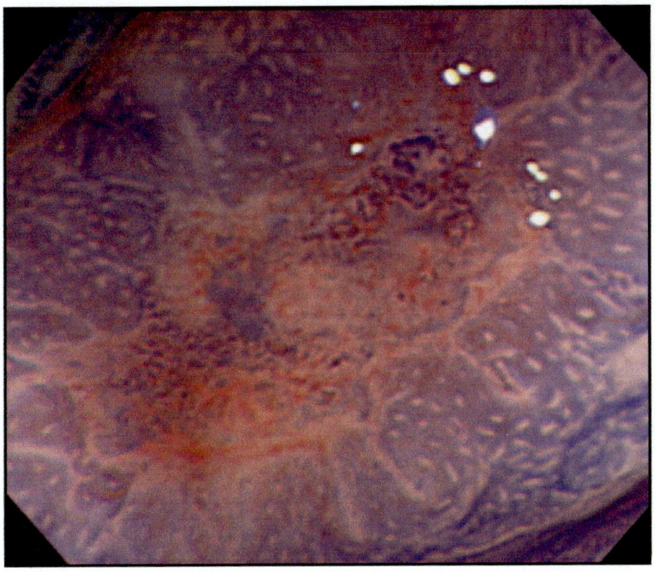

Figure 2-3. Magnification view of a depressed area after crystal violet dye stain. A fine dotted pit pattern (type III_S) is clearly seen.

Table 2-1. Kudo's Classification of Polyp Pit Patterns

TYPE	DESCRIPTION
Type I	Round, regular pits
Type II	Star-like pits
Type III_L	Tubular or roundish pits larger than type I
Type III_S	Small tubular or roundish pits smaller than type I
Type IV	Branched or gyrus-like pits
Type V_I	Markedly irregular pits
Type V_N	Nonstructural pits

More advanced lesions have higher numbered pit types, with type V lesions being most likely to harbor malignancy.

Information from Kudo S, Rubio CA, Teixeira CR, Kashida H, Kogure E. Pit pattern in colorectal neoplasia: endoscopic magnifying view. *Endoscopy.* 2001;33(4):367-373.

computer software processes the images after their natural acquisition (eg, i-Scan; Pentax Medical, and FICE; Fujifilm Corporation).[8,9] These types of imaging technologies are referred to as *virtual chromoendoscopy*.

Recent developments in magnification technology have proved to be significant additions for advanced imaging of gastrointestinal mucosa. One such development is confocal laser endomicroscopy (CLE),[10] which can be integrated within the endoscope itself (eCLE; Pentax Medical)[11] or probe based via a device passed through the endoscope's working channel (pCLE; Mauna-Kea Technologies).[12] These technologies require contrast enhancement by intravenously administered fluorescein dye, allowing in vivo

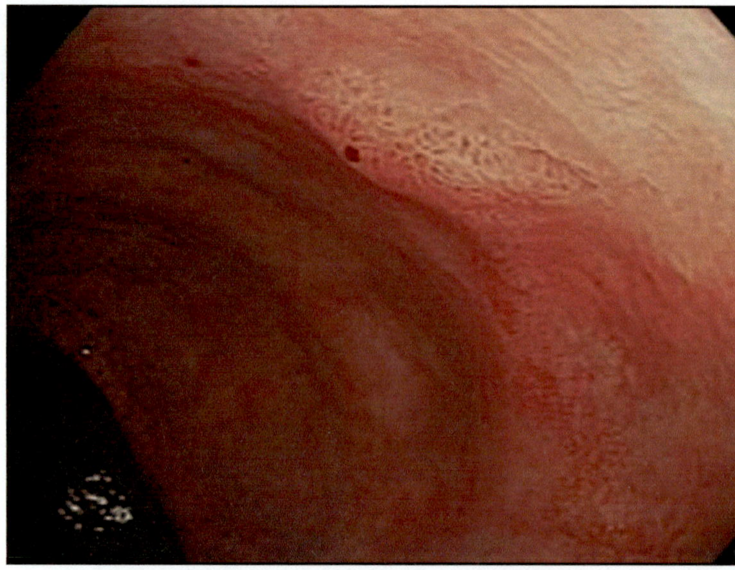

Figure 2-4. The mucosal pattern was slightly abnormal in this patient with longstanding ulcerative colitis (UC).

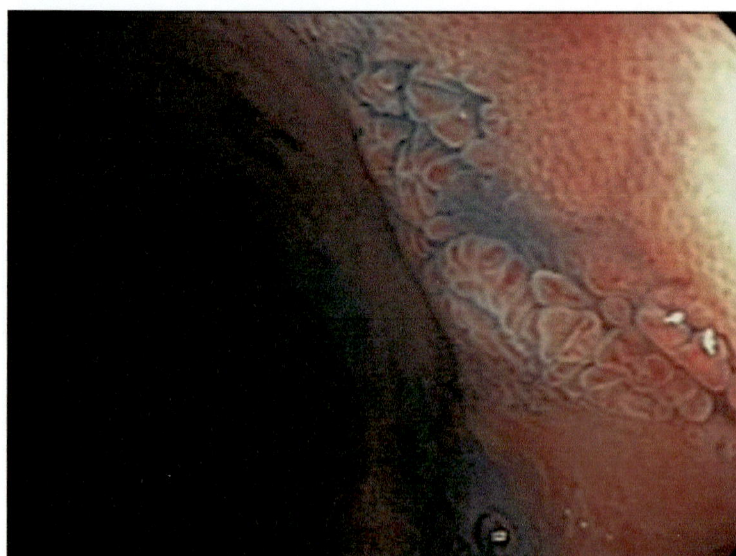

Figure 2-5. Chromoendoscopy with indigo carmine dye spray was performed to visualize the mucosal pattern of the same lesion in Figure 2-4.

cellular-level examination of tissue structures (ie, glandular and vascular structures). These technologies are often referred to as *virtual histology*, with a field of view of 475 μm (eCLE) or 240 μm (pCLE). Another virtual histology technology not yet approved by the US Food and Drug Administration is the Endocytoscopy System (Olympus America, Inc),[13] which uses methylene blue as an adjunct to detailed high-resolution white-light visualization.

One newly released endoscope system (EVIS EXERA III; Olympus America, Inc) features a dual-focus mechanism that incorporates a new near-focus mode, allowing the operator to visualize the surface closely. Magnification of the surface image by as much as nearly 45 times is possible, making this a significant enhancement to standard endoscopy. It should be noted that, although impressive, this magnification is less than that afforded

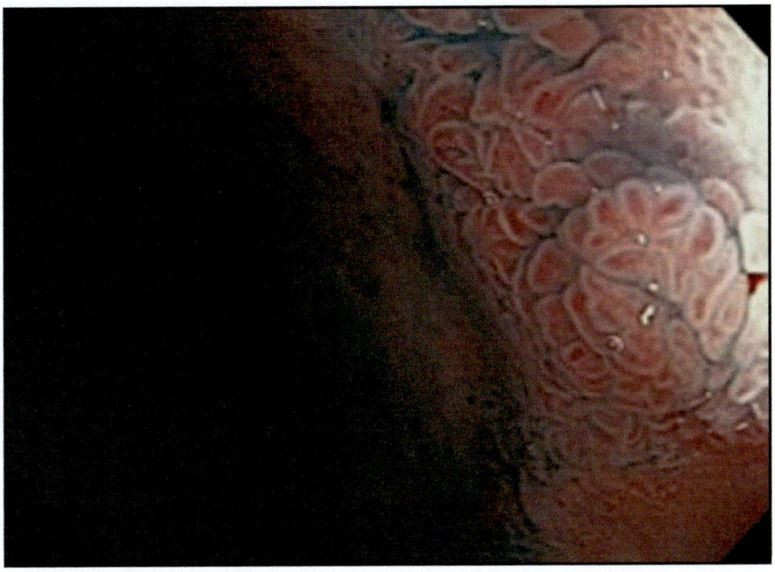

Figure 2-6. In the same lesion shown in Figure 2-5, an enlarged and thick tubular pit became apparent, suggestive of dysplastic mucosa.

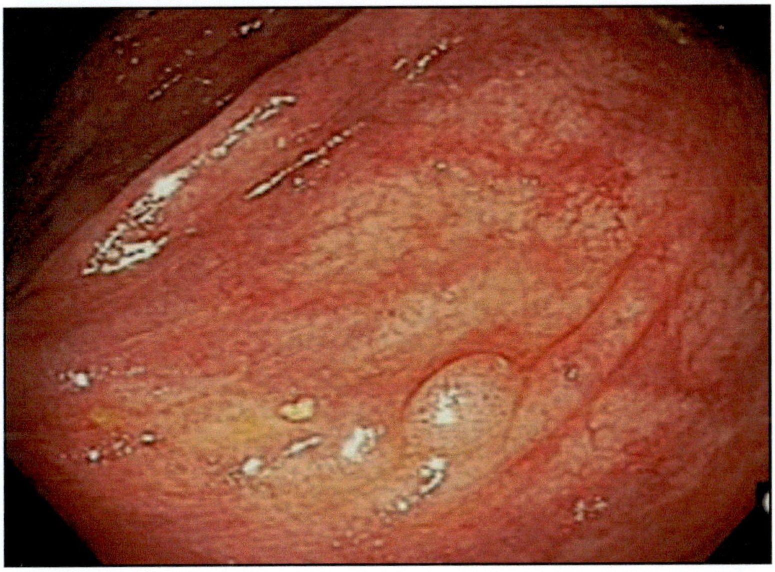

Figure 2-7. A commonly found small sessile polyp is seen with the use of white-light endoscopy.

by traditional magnification endoscopy, which can be as much as 150 times (Figures 2-9 and 2-10).[14]

All enhanced imaging techniques require excellent preparation of the colon for adequate colonoscopic examination. Further removal of any residual surface feces or mucus is essential for one to view the surface details (Figures 2-11 to 2-13). Once the surface is cleaned thoroughly, high-quality regular endoscopic visual inspection is necessary to characterize the lesion and identify the focus of interest (eg, a polyp, an area of suspected high-grade dysplasia, or invasive cancer). For dye-based techniques, contrast dye then is sprayed to enhance the pattern of the lesion, focusing on the area of concern as well as the margin of the lesion (Figure 2-14). For optimum visualization, each available dye requires slightly different steps after it is sprayed, which will be discussed in more depth later in this chapter.

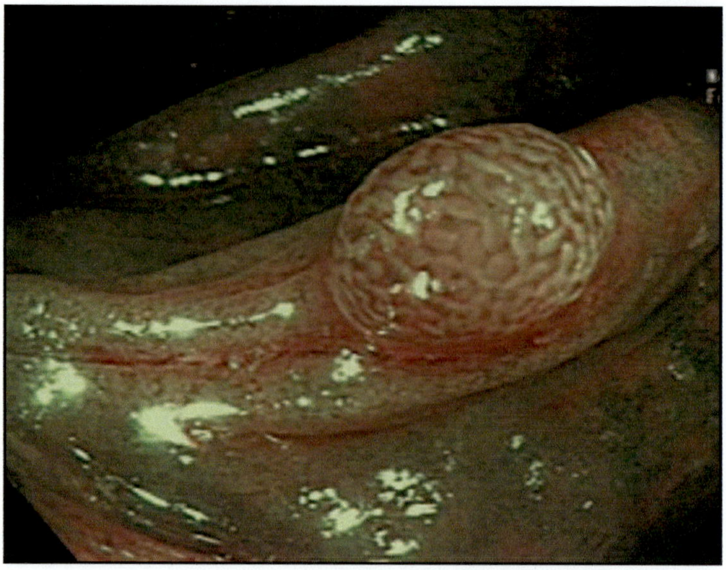

Figure 2-8. NBI chromoendoscopy of the same polyp seen in Figure 2-7, with a closer view showing a tubular pit pattern (pit type III_L).

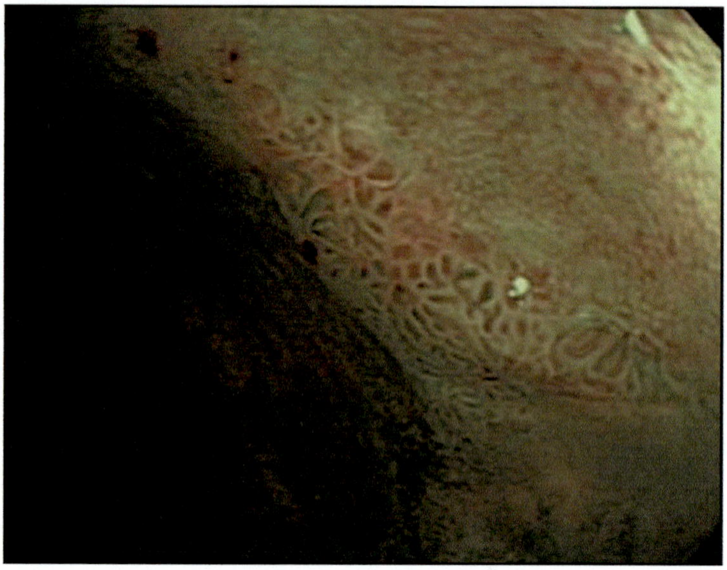

Figure 2-9. NBI image of the dysplastic change on the mucosa in a patient with longstanding UC (see Figures 2-4 to 2-6).

Enhanced Imaging Techniques: What They Can and Cannot Do

Chromoendoscopy and enhanced imaging have important roles in categorizing lesions into the subclassifications of colorectal neoplasms (eg, hyperplastic polyp, tubular adenoma, villous adenoma, adenoma with high-grade dysplasia, or invasive adenocarcinoma). They were expected to enhance detection ability for colorectal lesions, although largely this has not proved to be the case because most polypoid colorectal lesions are still found during high-resolution white-light endoscopic (WLE) examination, regardless of the use of enhanced imaging techniques. Therefore, the added benefit of these techniques is

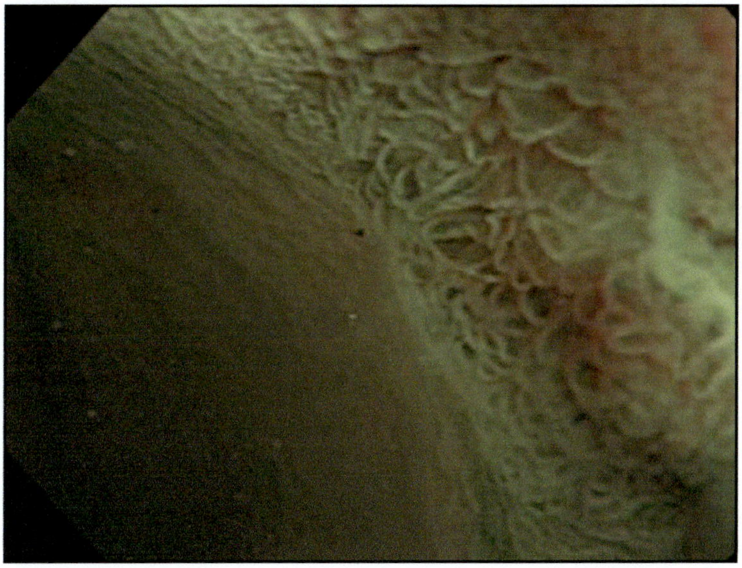

Figure 2-10. Near focus is used, and a magnified view is achieved. Details of the dysplastic surface pattern are seen clearly with a magnified view. The tubular and somewhat torturous pit pattern (type III_L and IV) is significantly larger than the normal pit pattern (type I) surrounding the abnormality (NICE classification type 2).

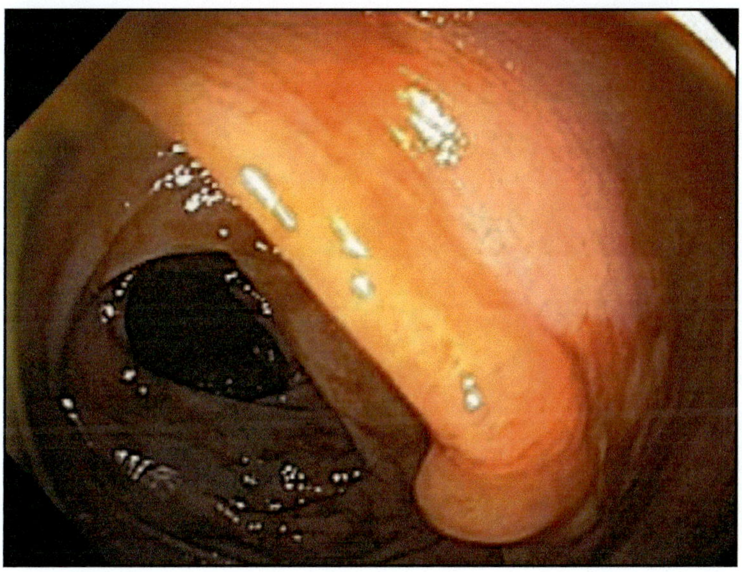

Figure 2-11. White-light image of a mucus-covered sessile polyp. The surface pattern is not seen clearly because of mucus.

mostly seen in the detection of flat, small, or hyperplastic lesions, and their overall benefit regarding polyp detection and cancer prevention over the long term is unclear.[15,16] This finding is similar to that of the new NBI technology, which does not provide a clear benefit in reducing the adenoma miss rate.[17,18]

The prediction of the actual histologic finding of colonic polyps by advanced imaging techniques is an exciting concept that could allow endoscopists to decide, in real time, which polyps to remove and which polyps could possibly be ignored. The use of indigo carmine chromoendoscopy to determine polyp type was recently reported to have a sensitivity of 82% to 95% and specificity of 64% to 95%.[2,19] This is encouraging but appears to be suboptimal when compared with the gold standard of histology. Refinements to this technique and increased operator experience may help improve these results in the future.

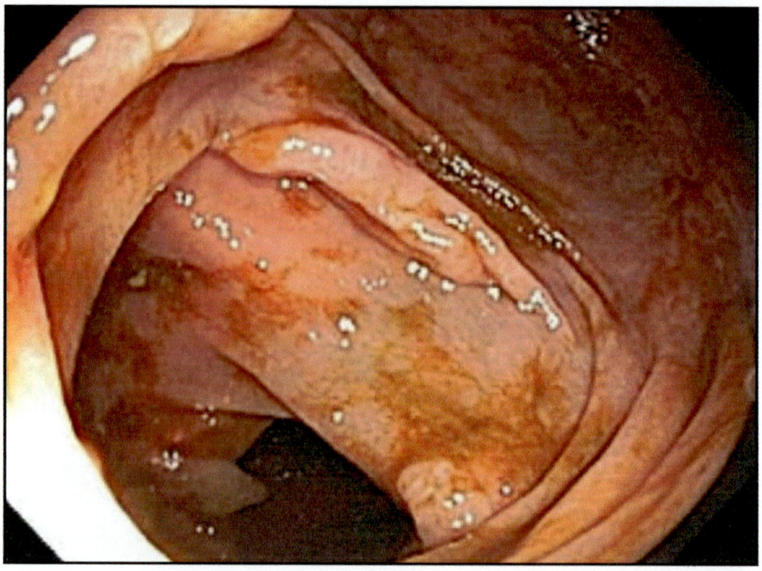

Figure 2-12. Same polyp as seen in Figure 2-11. Repeated irrigation with water revealed a normal pinkish color and slight increase in vascular pattern in the long view.

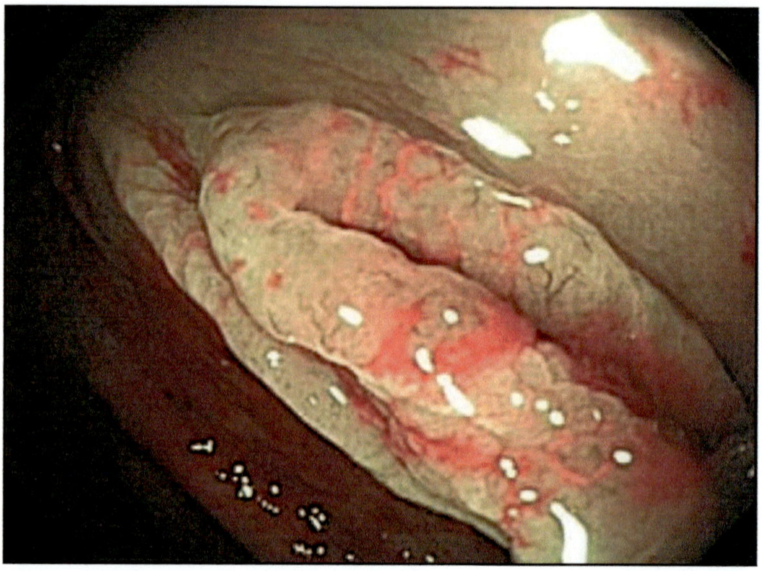

Figure 2-13. Near-focus view with NBI shows more details of the vascular pattern (prominent branched and torturous vessels) with enlarged pits without interference of overlying mucus.

To incorporate the enhanced vascular pattern seen with NBI, the Narrow Band Imaging International Colorectal Endoscopic (NICE) classification system was proposed.[20] Although subsequent study showed that this classification was useful for identifying deep submucosal invasion within lesions,[21] further study is needed. Also under investigation is magnification endoscopy, which may play a role in increasing the accuracy of determining polyp type.[22,23]

Magnification endoscopy is frequently used to obtain a clear view of portions of larger lesions. As such, it should be emphasized that the primary high-quality overview inspection available with high-resolution endoscopy is important in identifying the most concerning area within lesions. Once the area of greatest concern in a lesion has been identified, further inspection can be performed with enhanced imaging techniques (eg, chromoendoscopy or CLE) to solidify the findings. Still, similar to other advanced

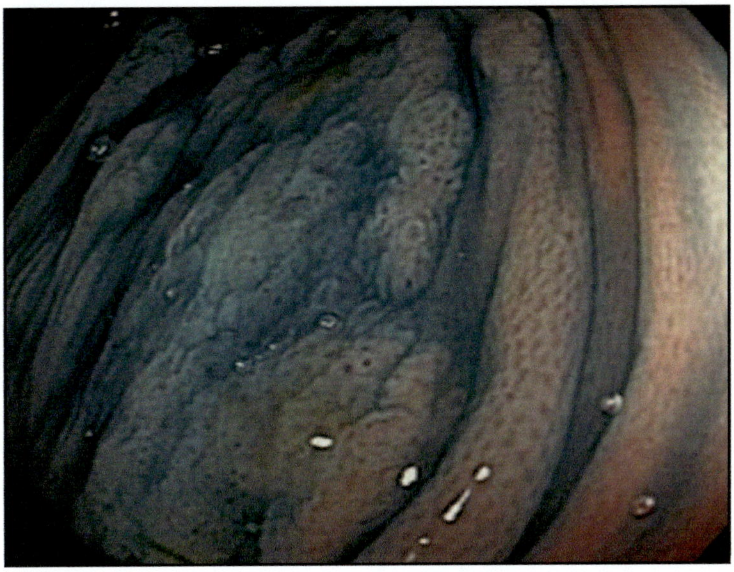

Figure 2-14. Indigo carmine chromoendoscopy clearly shows the margin of the lesion with a clear separation of the enlarged pits from ordinary pits.

techniques, magnification endoscopy remains an investigational adjunct in most contexts to supplement the daily colonoscopic practice.

When to Use Advanced Imaging Techniques

Large sessile (larger than 1 cm), flat, or depressed lesions are examined best with the addition of chromoendoscopy if their appearance is concerning or their borders are unclear. Small polyps (smaller than 1 cm) without nodularity, redness, a depressed area, or spontaneous bleeding are unlikely to be advanced neoplasia, and chromoendoscopy can be used to confirm the presence or, more likely, the absence of features of advanced neoplasia. Typically, virtual chromoendoscopy is more readily available (by the push of a button on the endoscope) and is used more easily to predict various histologic types for low-risk lesions than the dye spray method.

The dye spray method is most useful in the surveillance of IBD, most commonly chronic UC. It is now well accepted that chromoendoscopy improves detection of dysplastic changes in the colon of patients who have UC.[6,24-26] In 2004, Kiesslich and Neurath[27] suggested the SURFACE guidelines (strict patient selection, unmask mucosal changes, reduce peristalsis, full-length staining of the colon [panchromoendoscopy], augmented detection with dyes, crypt analysis, and endoscopically targeted biopsies) to maximize the utility of chromoendoscopy in patients with UC, and either targeted or pancolonic staining can be used. These guidelines provide a rationale and overview of the technique.

Step-by-Step Instructions for Advanced Imaging Techniques

Identification of concerning lesions under a regular or high-definition (HD) WLE view is the first step (ie, one first must identify a target for advanced imaging using standard imaging techniques). Irrigation of the area should be performed to clear any remaining mucus or fecal material (see Figures 2-11 to 2-13.) The area is examined closely to confirm the presence of the lesion, and then it is studied thoroughly to identify any concerning features such as excessive redness, nodularity, a depressed area, or ulceration, all of which suggest more advanced dysplasia or neoplasia within the lesion. The area with the most advanced dysplasia should be the target area for further detailed examination with the following advanced techniques.

Targeted Chromoendoscopy

After the lesion is cleared of any surface debris and a thorough regular WLE examination has been performed, one then can spray the dye solution (typically indigo carmine 0.2% to 0.8% solution) directly through the working channel or endoscope or with a dedicated spray catheter. One should wait a few seconds for the dye to settle along the surface of the mucosa, but excessive waiting is not needed because the dye only needs to effectively coat the surface of the mucosa. Immediate examination with near focus (if available) can be performed to determine the surface pattern (pit pattern classification).[3] Indigo carmine dye spray can be repeated as many times as needed because the dye tends to flow away or wash away easily.

For dedicated magnification endoscopy, crystal violet (0.05% to 0.1% solution) can be sprayed gently to stain the surface (see Figures 2-1 to 2-3). This technique is best for identifying types III_S and V pit patterns, but without dedicated magnification endoscopy, this dye is not necessary or useful.

Targeted Virtual Chromoendoscopy

After the initial steps explained previously are completed, virtual chromoendoscopy is activated with the push of a button in any endoscopic system. Once the imaging modality is activated, closer visualization is performed, with particular attention to pit pattern as well as vascular structures, which are often enhanced to visualize the pattern. One company, Olympus America Inc, offers a near-view mode integrated into certain endoscopes to allow a closer view that is equal to the moderate magnification view. One can switch between WLE and virtual chromoendoscopic images for comparison or to facilitate normal maneuvers under white light to reposition the endoscope tip against the lesions or to further irrigate lesions. A distal attachment cap or hood may be used to maintain the distance from the lens to the target lesion for maximal view during a close-up or magnification. If a cap or hood is not available, an endoscopic accessory such as a snare or needle catheter can be used to maintain the distance between the endoscope and the target.

Virtual Histology

Virtual histology with CLE or endocytoscopy further limits the area of inspection in exchange for more magnified images. For confocal microscopy, the intravenous injection of fluorescein is necessary before visualization of the area. All equipment should be ready (CLE tower and probe or activation of CLE on the endoscope) before injection of the medication. Intravenous fluorescein is distributed throughout the vasculature within seconds and lasts as long as 30 minutes. Optimal visualization is usually achieved for the first 8 minutes after the drug is delivered. The usual dose is 2.5 to 5 mL of 10% fluorescein.[28]

Continuous visualization of the lesion, mostly at the focal area, should be performed promptly, and it should be recorded appropriately for later review and interpretation (either as a video clip or still images). The use of CLE is another situation where a distal attachment cap or hood may enhance the quality of acquired images because it maintains the distance while the area is scanned.

Screening and Surveillance for Dysplasia in Inflammatory Bowel Disease

Important steps to maximize chromoendoscopy findings were published as the SURFACE guidelines,[27] and these should be well understood. Dye spray with either 0.1% indigo carmine or 0.1% methylene blue is used to enhance the surface pattern. Methylene blue takes as long as 60 seconds to be absorbed, and the endoscopist needs to allow time for staining (continuous contact of the dye solution with the surface of the lesion). After adequate time has been allowed for HD WLE examination, segmental chromoendoscopy is performed, for which the use of a spray catheter is recommended to distribute the dye solution evenly over the large surface area that needs to be examined in patients with UC. Some studies have performed right- and left-segment chromoendoscopy (segmental examination separating at the end of transverse colon),[25] but shorter segments are usually recommended, alternating with HD WLE examination in 5- to 15-cm segments. Excess dye solution should be suctioned, and the examination should be performed from the proximal to the distal end of the colon segment of interest. The typical volume of methylene blue used for full colonoscopic surveillance of patients with UC is 60 to 100 mL. Any visible abnormality should be examined carefully with reference to its pit pattern and a biopsy performed, with specimens clearly labeled as to location of origin within the colon.

Avoiding Complications

Chromoendoscopy uses only dye spray in addition to standard endoscopic equipment and is considered nontoxic and extremely safe. Magnification endoscopy, however, has a minimal additional risk related to the use of fluorescein (1.4%). In rare cases, nausea, vomiting, and severe allergic reactions can develop in patients exposed to fluorescein dye.[28]

Advanced Tips

To evaluate lesions, especially with advanced imaging, it is of utmost importance to clean the surface first before any endoscopic examination is performed. Repeated water irrigation should be performed to clear any debris or mucus adhered to the lesion. Advanced neoplastic lesions tend to bleed when strongly irrigated by water jet; therefore, the strength of the water stream should be reduced at first, and then it can be increased as necessary. Use of spray catheters to deliver dye is recommended because they help distribute the dye evenly, minimizing pooling of excess dye. In addition, spray catheters can be used as an arm to hold down mucosal folds or to maintain a steady distance from the polyp for a near and magnified view to visualize the pattern in the most static manner

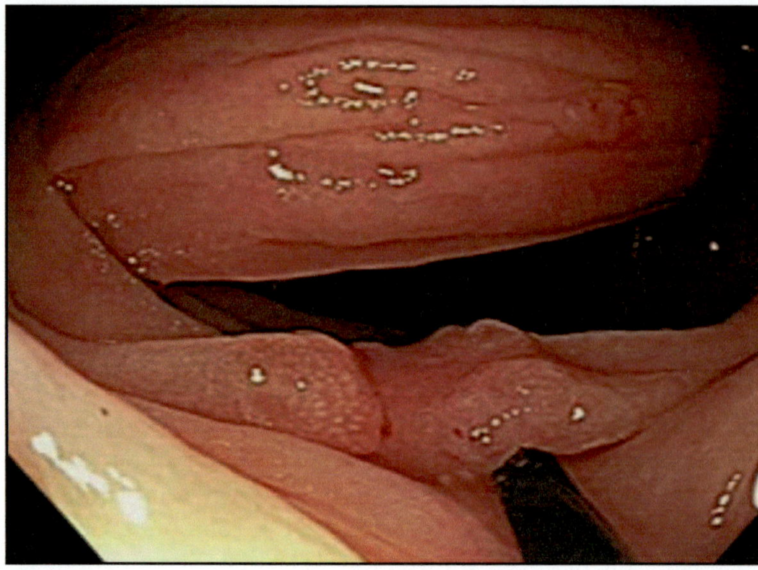

Figure 2-15. The sheath of the injection needle is used to expose a small lesion with the suspected depressed area (suspected advanced dysplasia or invasive cancer within the lesion).

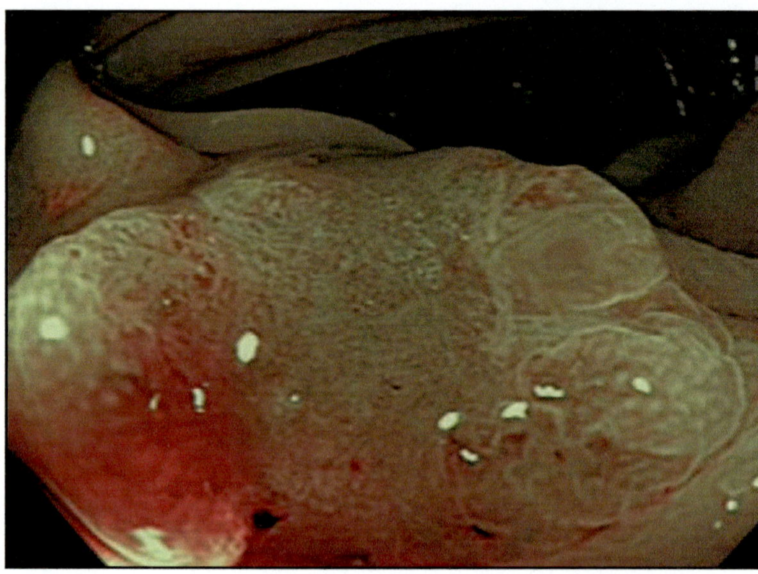

Figure 2-16. NBI with near focus shows the depressed area with irregular, nearly destructed pits (type V_I). The sheath of the needle will maintain the distance during examination of the pattern in detail.

possible (Figures 2-15 and 2-16). If spray catheters are not available, dye delivery with a simple syringe (injecting through the working channel of the endoscope) works well in most situations. The addition of 5 mL of dye solution to a 20-mL syringe (15 cc of air) is the most commonly used formulation. Stronger dye solutions tend to interfere with examination, especially if excessive amounts are sprayed. Generally, it is advised that one use diluted dye concentrations first to evaluate the effect of revealing important surface patterns before moving on to stronger dye solutions.

Conclusion

Although WLE examination remains the mainstay for endoscopic evaluation of the colon, numerous enhanced imaging techniques are available. These techniques provide a more focused and enhanced view of colonic mucosa and lesions, which can aid in the identification and assessment of polyps or other areas of concern, facilitating the formulation of individualized, comprehensive plans for endoscopic and medical or surgical treatment. Further developments in this area are ongoing to help refine which technique is best suited for specific situations.

Acknowledgment

The author would like to express his sincere appreciation to Alissa Bults, MS, for her exceptional assistance in preparing this chapter.

References

1. Tada M, Katoh S, Kohli Y, Kawai K. On the dye spraying method in colonofiberscopy. *Endoscopy.* 1977;8(2):70-74.
2. Wong Kee Song LM, Adler DC, ASGE Technology Committee, et al. Chromoendoscopy. *Gastrointest Endosc.* 2007;66(4):639-649.
3. Kudo S, Rubio CA, Teixeira CR, Kashida H, Kogure E. Pit pattern in colorectal neoplasia: endoscopic magnifying view. *Endoscopy.* 2001;33(4):367-373.
4. Kudo S, Hirota S, Nakajima T, et al. Colorectal tumors and pit pattern. *J Clin Pathol.* 1994;47(10):880-885.
5. Matsuda T, Fujii T, Saito Y, et al. Efficacy of the invasive/non-invasive pattern by magnifying chromoendoscopy to estimate the depth of invasion of early colorectal neoplasms. *Am J Gastroenterol.* 2008;103(11):2700-2706.
6. Kiesslich R, Neurath MF. Chromoendoscopy in inflammatory bowel disease. *Gastroenterol Clin North Am.* 2012;41(2):291-302.
7. Machida H, Sano Y, Hamamoto Y, et al. Narrow-band imaging in the diagnosis of colorectal mucosal lesions: a pilot study. *Endoscopy.* 2004;36(12):1094-1098.
8. Hoffman A, Sar F, Goetz M, et al. High definition colonoscopy combined with i-Scan is superior in the detection of colorectal neoplasias compared with standard video colonoscopy: a prospective randomized controlled trial. *Endoscopy.* 2010;42(10):827-833.
9. Pohl J, May A, Rabenstein T, Pech O, Ell C. Computed virtual chromoendoscopy: a new tool for enhancing tissue surface structures. *Endoscopy.* 2007;39(1):80-83.
10. Neumann H, Kiesslich R, Wallace MB, Neurath MF. Confocal laser endomicroscopy: technical advances and clinical applications. *Gastroenterology.* 2010;139(2):388-392, 392.e1-2.
11. Kiesslich R, Burg J, Vieth M, et al. Confocal laser endoscopy for diagnosing intraepithelial neoplasias and colorectal cancer in vivo. *Gastroenterology.* 2004;127(3):706-713.
12. Wallace MB, Fockens P. Probe-based confocal laser endomicroscopy. *Gastroenterology.* 2009;136(5): 1509-1513.
13. Kwon RS, Wong Kee Song LM, ASGE Technology Committee, et al. Endocytoscopy. *Gastrointest Endosc.* 2009;70(4):610-613.
14. Kwon RS, Adler DG, ASGE Technology Committee, et al. High-resolution and high-magnification endoscopes. *Gastrointest Endosc.* 2009;69(3, pt 1):399-407.
15. Brooker JC, Saunders BP, Shah SG, et al. Total colonic dye-spray increases the detection of diminutive adenomas during routine colonoscopy: a randomized controlled trial. *Gastrointest Endosc.* 2002;56(3):333-338.

16. Le Rhun M, Coron E, Parlier D, et al. High resolution colonoscopy with chromoscopy versus standard colonoscopy for the detection of colonic neoplasia: a randomized study. *Clin Gastroenterol Hepatol.* 2006;4(3):349-354.
17. Dinesen L, Chua TJ, Kaffes AJ. Meta-analysis of narrow-band imaging versus conventional colonoscopy for adenoma detection. *Gastrointest Endosc.* 2012;75(3):604-611.
18. Kaltenbach T, Friedland S, Soetikno R. A randomised tandem colonoscopy trial of narrow band imaging versus white light examination to compare neoplasia miss rates. *Gut.* 2008;57(10):1406-1412.
19. Eisen GM, Kim CY, Fleischer DE, et al. High-resolution chromoendoscopy for classifying colonic polyps: a multicenter study. *Gastrointest Endosc.* 2002;55(6):687-694.
20. Tanaka S, Sano Y. Aim to unify the narrow band imaging (NBI) magnifying classification for colorectal tumors: current status in Japan from a summary of the consensus symposium in the 79th Annual Meeting of the Japan Gastroenterological Endoscopy Society. *Dig Endosc.* 2011;23 Suppl 1:131-139.
21. Hayashi N, Tanaka S, Hewett DG, et al. Endoscopic prediction of deep submucosal invasive carcinoma: validation of the Narrow-Band Imaging International Colorectal Endoscopic (NICE) classification. *Gastrointest Endosc.* 2013;78(4):625-632.
22. Yoshida N, Yagi N, Yanagisawa A, Naito Y. Image-enhanced endoscopy for diagnosis of colorectal tumors in view of endoscopic treatment. *World J Gastroenterol.* 2012;4(12):545-555.
23. Fu KI, Sano Y, Kato S, et al. Chromoendoscopy using indigo carmine dye spraying with magnifying observation is the most reliable method for differential diagnosis between non-neoplastic and neoplastic colorectal lesions: a prospective study. *Endoscopy.* 2004;36(12):1089-1093.
24. Rutter MD, Saunders BP, Schofield G, Forbes A, Price AB, Talbot IC. Pancolonic indigo carmine dye spraying for the detection of dysplasia in ulcerative colitis. *Gut.* 2004;53(2):256-260.
25. Marion JF, Waye JD, Present DH, et al. Chromoendoscopy-targeted biopsies are superior to standard colonoscopic surveillance for detecting dysplasia in inflammatory bowel disease patients: a prospective endoscopic trial. *Am J Gastroenterol.* 2008;103(9):2342-2349.
26. Subramanian V, Mannath J, Raguath K, Hawkey CH. Meta-analysis: the diagnostic yield of chromoendoscopy for detecting dysplasia in patients with colonic inflammatory bowel disease. *Aliment Pharmacol Ther.* 2011;33(3):304-312.
27. Kiesslich R, Neurath MF. Surveillance colonoscopy in ulcerative colitis: magnifying chromoendoscopy in the spotlight. *Gut.* 2004;53(2):165-167.
28. Wallace M, Meining A, Canto MI, et al. The safety of intravenous fluorescein for confocal laser endomicroscopy in the gastrointestinal tract. *Aliment Pharmacol Ther.* 2010;31(5):548-552.

Please visit www.routledge.com/9781617116148 to access additional material.

3

Air Versus Carbon Dioxide Insufflation Versus Water Immersion During Colonoscopy

Douglas Pleskow, MD, AGAF, FASGE; Tolga Erim, DO; and Gyanprakash Ketwaroo, MD

The colon is approximately 1.5 m long and, along with the small intestine and other organs, occupies a rather small space in the human body. Therefore, the colon is largely collapsed within the abdominal cavity most of the time. During colonoscopy, the colonic lumen must be distended enough to enable adequate visualization of the walls of the colon, but not so much as to cause significant pain or perforation from barotrauma. Colonoscopy with air insufflation is the standard technique and has been for many years (Figure 3-1).

However, there are several disadvantages to using air in colonoscopy. Air accumulates in the right colon during insertion and withdrawal of the colonoscope. This accumulation in the colon can cause significant discomfort during the procedure and recovery. The distention also causes elongation of the colon, which can make cecal intubation more challenging, especially in patients with a so-called *redundant colon*. The discomfort caused by the distention can lead to bearing down by the patient, stiffening the abdominal wall and making it more difficult to assist with external pressure in patients who are not deeply sedated.

The search for alternatives to air insufflation during colonoscopy has been driven by the benefits of unsedated or on-demand–sedation colonoscopy. Patients who have colonoscopy without sedation have a minimal recovery period, do not need a chaperone after the procedure, and can return to work or their daily activities (including driving an automobile) without delay. Furthermore, in unsedated patients, the oral preparation can be taken closer to the time of colonoscopy and there are no anesthesia-related side effects. The need for transportation and time off from work are both barriers to screening colonoscopy, and unsedated colonoscopy can potentially help reduce both.[1] In addition,

Adler DG, ed.
Core Concepts in Colonoscopy (pp 27-37).

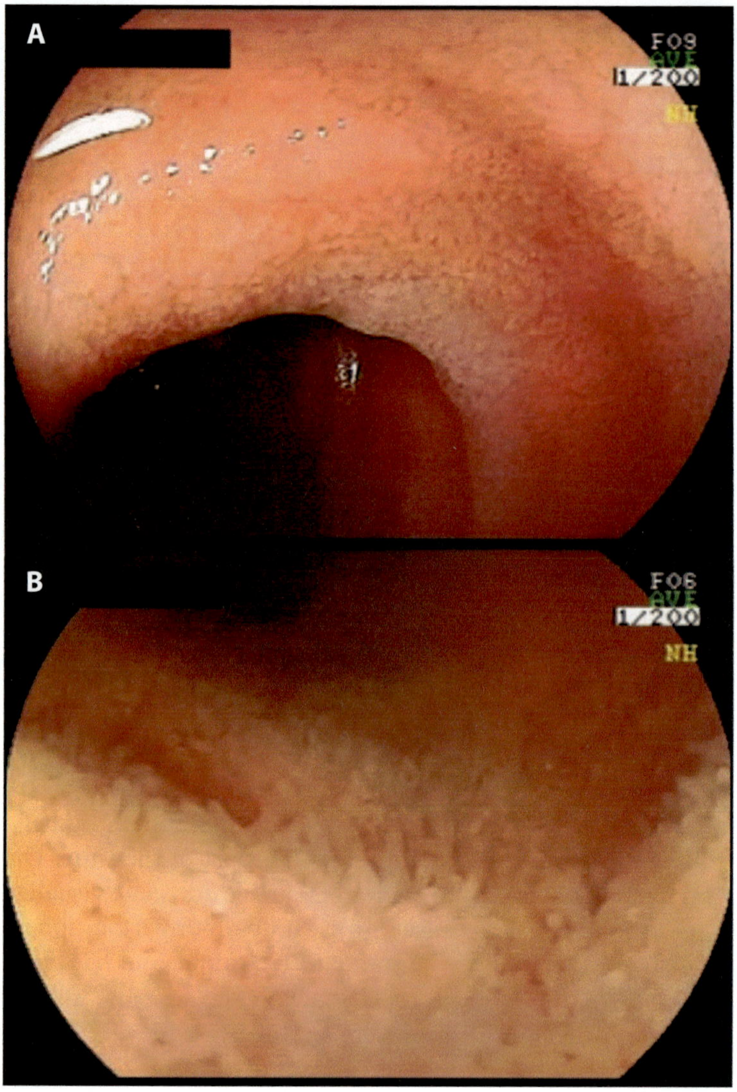

Figure 3-1. Typical endoscopic views of (A) the colon and (B) the terminal ileum when using air insufflation.

anesthesia assistance in colonoscopy has been associated with increased overall complications in some populations, especially the risk of aspiration.[2]

To that end, water and carbon dioxide have been proposed as substitutes for air insufflation. The advantage of colonoscopy with air insufflation, when compared with colonoscopy with carbon dioxide and/or water, is that air is readily available in abundance and is less costly because it does not require additional equipment to obtain or store room air. Air and carbon dioxide distend the bowel and thus create a clear path for mucosal visualization. Water also distends the bowel but can mix with stool and thus worsen visualization in patients who have had suboptimal preparation.[3]

The aim of studies evaluating the use of carbon dioxide and water in patients undergoing colonoscopy has primarily been to demonstrate their relative advantages over air insufflation while still achieving the same quality and outcomes. The studies mainly have concentrated on pain, adenoma detection rate, and cecal intubation rate.

Water Assistance in Colonoscopy

Baumann[4] first described using water instillation to aid in traversing the sigmoid colon in 1999. Instilling 200 mL water into the first bend of the sigmoid colon shortened insertion time by 31%. The first randomized, controlled trial of water-assisted colonoscopy was performed in 2002 by Hamamoto et al.[5] In this study, 500 to 1000 mL of water was instilled into the colon by enema at the start of the procedure. The results were shorter insertion time, less pain, and similar cecal intubation and disease detection rates when compared with colonoscopy with air insufflation. These methods of using water as needed in combination with air is sometimes referred to as *air-water hybrid*.[6]

The current phase of water-assisted colonoscopy research was sparked by several recent studies, starting with a 2007 study by Leung et al[7] noting that 52% of patients at a Veterans Affairs Medical Center in the United States were able to complete their colonoscopy with on-demand sedation and warm water infusion. Two main variations on water-assisted colonoscopy have been developed since then: water immersion and water exchange. Water immersion is the standard water-based technique where water is infused into the colon during insertion and suctioned predominantly during withdrawal (Figure 3-2). The water exchange method was developed later to decrease discomfort caused by the large volume of water infused into the colon. In water exchange, the water is infused into and then suctioned out of the colon predominantly during the insertion. Although there has not been a head-to-head comparison of these 2 techniques, the water-exchange method has been found to reduce pain scores 50% to 68% vs 7.7% to 35% with the water-immersion method.[8]

There is no consensus on the appropriate temperature for the water that is to be infused into the patient. Studies have used cold water, water judged to be warm to the touch, or water kept at 37°C via a water bath. A recent study found no difference in the amount of sedation needed with warm or cold water, arguing against a clear winner in this debate.[9]

The infusion of water may be accomplished with a syringe of water or by attaching a catheter connected to a dedicated water pump through the biopsy channel of the colonoscope (Figure 3-3). Newer colonoscopes have a dedicated water-infusion channel that also can be connected to a water pump. The amount of water infused varies from 200 mL in a well-prepared colon to as much as 2 L in a suboptimally prepared colon. As the colonoscope is advanced, any pockets of air can be suctioned out. Water is infused to identify and open the lumen. As areas of angulation are encountered, the tip of the colonoscope is directed toward the lumen, and infused water spreads the collapsed mucosal folds apart in a manner similar to that used in air insufflation colonoscopy. Any residual stool can be suctioned as encountered, and clean water is infused repeatedly to keep the visual field clear. External pressure and position changes are used as in air insufflation colonoscopy to assist in cecal intubation. Cecal intubation is confirmed by air insufflation and visualization of the appendiceal orifice and ileocecal valve.[10]

As with all endoscopic techniques, there is a learning curve to the water-assisted method. One study demonstrated that the cecal intubation rate approaches the standard air colonoscopy rate after 75 to 100 cases.[11] The most common reason for failure to achieve cecal intubation with the water method was misidentification of the cecum. The mean insertion time for water-assisted colonoscopy is 5 to 13 minutes in experienced hands.[8]

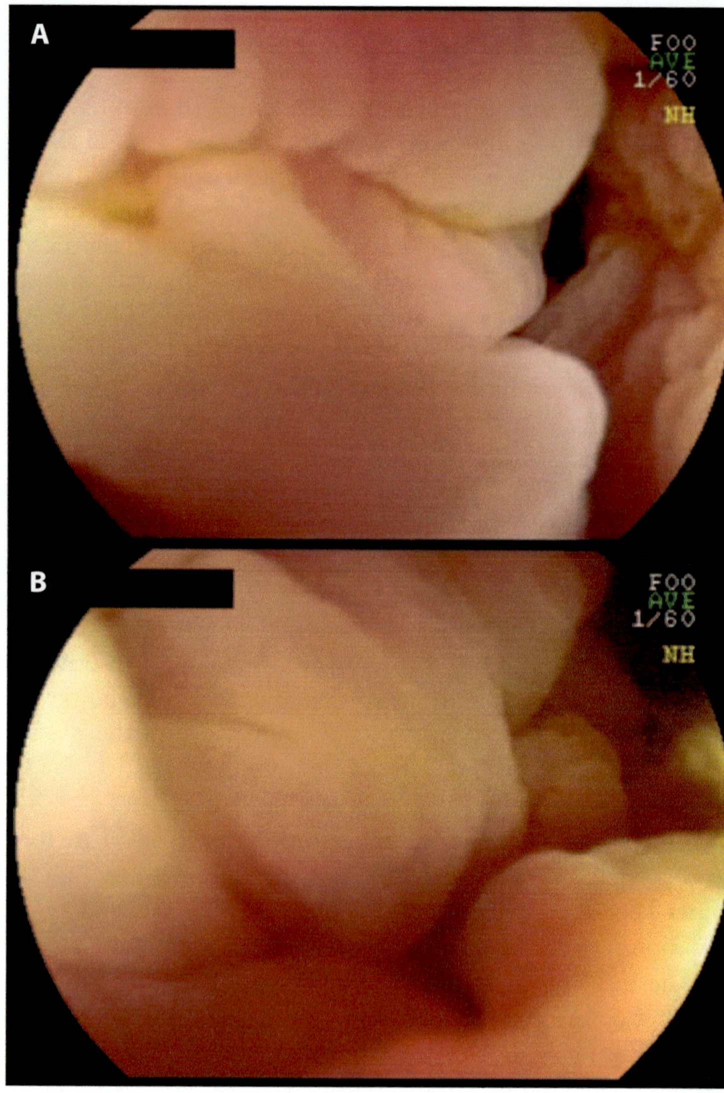

Figure 3-2. (A and B) Representative images of the colon during insertion of the colonoscope during water-assisted colonoscopy.

Water infusion during colonoscopy has been found to significantly reduce pain and the need for sedation and/or medication doses without adversely affecting the cecal intubation rate, insertion time, and disease/polyp detection rate.[12,13] Early studies noted a lower cecal intubation rate with water infusion colonoscopy, but this was found to normalize when air insufflation could be used as needed.[13] Some data suggest that water infusion reduces the need for position change and straightening maneuvers in patients who have had an incomplete colonoscopy in the past.[14] It has been postulated that water-assisted colonoscopy may minimize the need for these techniques by minimizing colonic lengthening during the procedure (as commonly occurs with air and carbon dioxide insufflation).[15] As such, water-exchange colonoscopy may be useful in achieving cecal intubation in patients who are anticipated to have difficult colonoscopies, such as those with prior failed attempts at cecal intubation or those who have had prior abdominal or pelvic surgery.[16]

Water-assisted colonoscopy has been found to be helpful in regard to polyp detection and resection. It has been noted that there is an optical zoom effect that takes place when

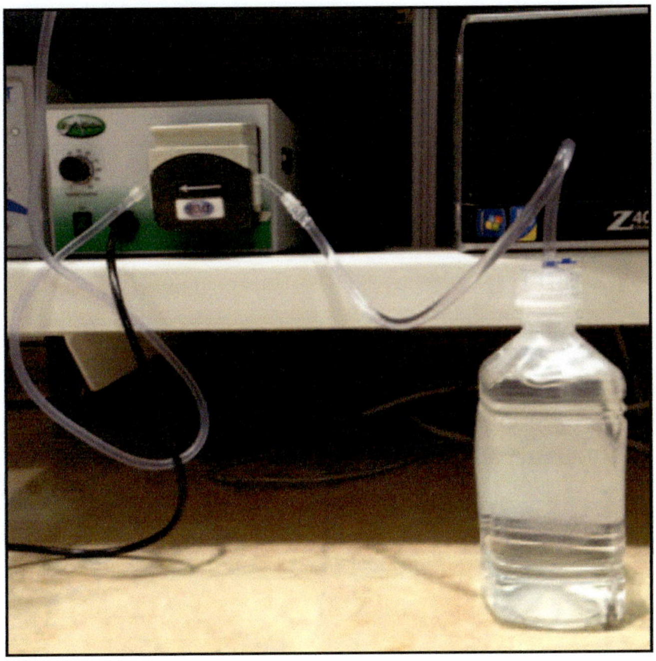

Figure 3-3. Typical appearance of a colonoscopic water pump and disposable water bottle.

the mucosa is viewed under water and the character of the mucosal surface is differentiated more easily, in a manner somewhat analogous to the oil immersion effect seen in microscopy.[17,18] Submucosal injection often is used during polypectomy and endoscopic mucosal resection to reduce the risks of unintentional muscularis propria resection and perforation. It has been proposed that water distention of the colon creates a buoyancy effect, whereby adenomatous tissue floats rather than being compressed by the expansile pressure of the air insufflation, thus potentially obviating the need for submucosal injection in some patients. Water immersion may also be helpful in patients with lower gastrointestinal bleeding because it can assist in identifying sites of active bleeding (Figure 3-4).[19] With air insufflation, blood often pools over the bleeding source and can make identification of sites for treatment difficult. Water infusion prevents pooling of blood and often highlights the exact site of ongoing blood loss because blood usually floats away to reveal, rather than obscure, the source. Control of bleeding with clipping, cautery, and even argon plasma coagulation with direct contact can be performed while the bleeding site is submerged under water.[18]

Carbon Dioxide-Assisted Colonoscopy

Although widely used for decades, air insufflation during colonoscopy is not without drawbacks, some of which have already been discussed. In the early days of colonoscopy, there was also concern regarding the potential for explosions to occur during the use of electrocautery in the setting of air insufflation, especially in patients with a suboptimally prepared colon. Carbon dioxide was proposed as a safe alternative to air because of its noncombustible nature. Experience has shown that colonoscopic explosions are exceptionally rare in practice, and air has proved to be safe on the whole. Surprisingly, initial

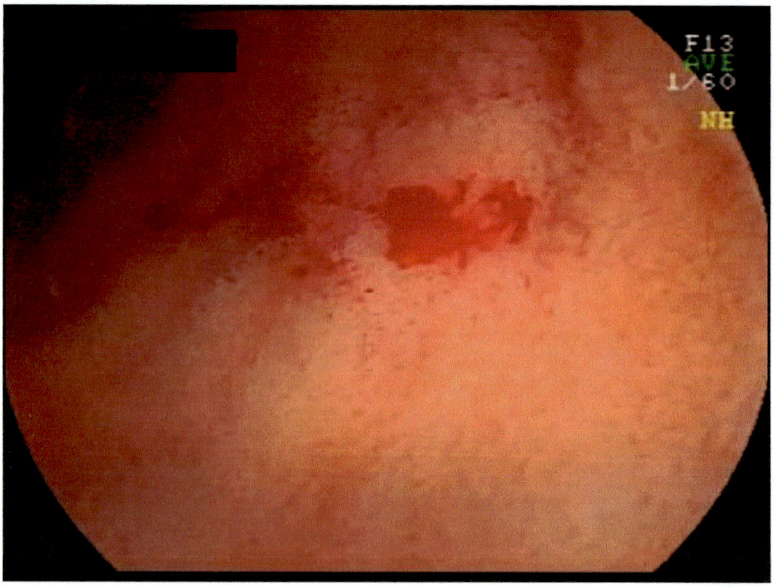

Figure 3-4. Source of active bleeding identified in the colon during water-assisted colonoscopy.

studies using carbon dioxide for insufflation showed other unexpected benefits, including enhanced colonic blood flow, reduced pain, and faster recovery times.[20]

The technique of carbon dioxide–assisted colonoscopy is largely identical to standard air insufflation colonoscopy. This is a major advantage when considering the learning curve necessary for water-assisted colonoscopy; carbon dioxide–assisted colonoscopy essentially has no learning curve for experienced endoscopists.

Carbon dioxide–assisted colonoscopy does require the use of additional hardware in the form of an external carbon dioxide tank and pump, which must be connected to the endoscope via tubing (Figures 3-5 and 3-6).

Of critical importance is the fact that carbon dioxide is absorbed quickly from the colon into the bloodstream and removed from the body via exhalation. Carbon dioxide–assisted colonoscopy does increase the end-tidal carbon dioxide level of the patient, but this is almost always of no clinical relevance.

Initial studies of carbon dioxide–assisted colonoscopy focused on the volume of gas needed for adequate insufflation. In an early study by Bretthauer et al,[21] gas volumes used during the procedure were measured in 249 patients having screening colonoscopy with either air or carbon dioxide. There was no statistically significant difference in either the mean total volume of gas used or the rate of insufflation of carbon dioxide or air during these colonoscopies. Patients tended to require approximately 8 L of gas at a rate of approximately 250 mL/min.[21]

The rapid absorption of carbon dioxide directly results in less retention of gas in the patient after colonoscopy. In a small study by Stevenson et al,[22] 56 patients were assigned randomly to receive colonoscopy with either air or carbon dioxide insufflation, and gas retention was measured by abdominal radiograph 1 hour after the procedure. Ninety-four percent of patients with carbon dioxide insufflation retained trace to minimal colonic gas, whereas 96% of patients receiving air had air in the whole colon or had more significant colonic distention, including 18% with a maximum colonic diameter greater than 10 cm.[22] This correlated with significantly reduced pain in the carbon dioxide–insufflation group compared with the air-insufflation group at 6 hours (3% vs 50%; $P = .0005$) and 24 hours

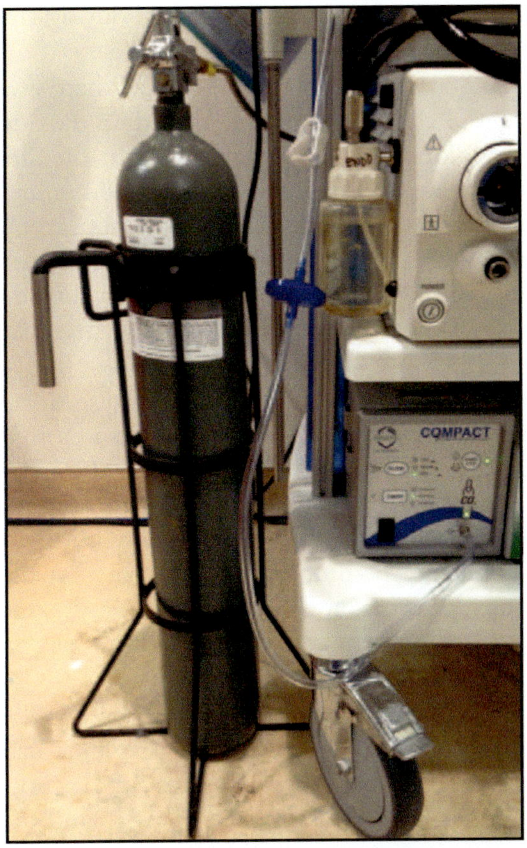

Figure 3-5. Carbon dioxide tank used for carbon dioxide–assisted colonoscopy.

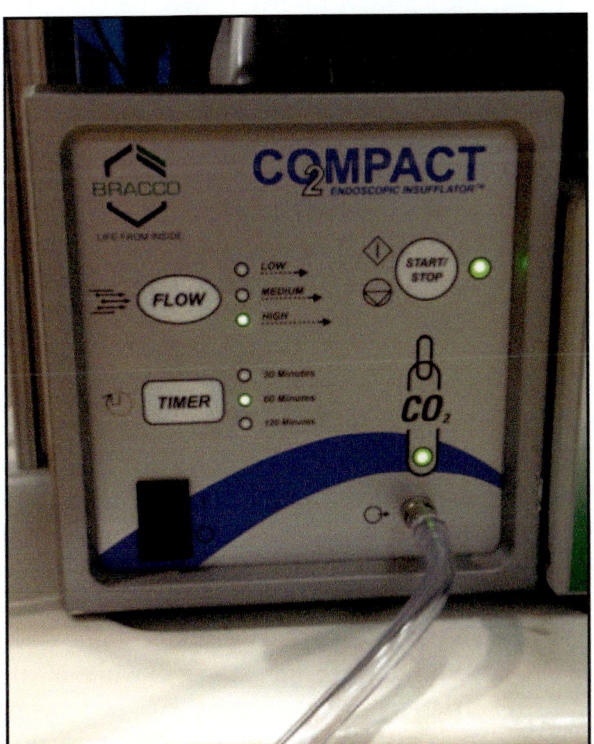

Figure 3-6. Representative commercially available pump for carbon dioxide.

(5% vs 36%, $P = .01$) postprocedure. There was no difference in reported pain during the procedure with either method.

In a larger study of carbon dioxide–assisted colonoscopy by Sumanac et al,[23] there was significantly reduced postprocedure colonic gas and abdominal pain with carbon dioxide insufflation compared with air. One hour after colonoscopy, 71% of patients in the air-insufflation group had a colonic diameter greater than 6 cm as measured on abdominal radiograph, compared with only 6% of patients in the carbon dioxide–insufflation group ($P < .0001$). Forty-five percent of patients receiving air insufflation had mild to moderate pain 1 hour after colonoscopy compared with 7% of patients receiving carbon dioxide ($P < .0001$). There were similar reports of pain in both groups immediately after the procedure.[23]

Some investigators have hypothesized that insufflation with carbon dioxide during withdrawal may have the most benefit. In a recent study of 100 patients by Hsu et al,[24] patients were randomly assigned to 3 groups: 33 patients received air insufflation throughout colonoscopy, 33 patients received carbon dioxide insufflation only during withdrawal, and 34 patients received carbon dioxide insufflation during both insertion and withdrawal. In this study, pain scores were similarly low during the procedure in all arms. At the end of colonoscopy and 1 hour after colonoscopy, both groups receiving carbon dioxide had a statistically significant decrease in pain. However, the pain scores in both carbon dioxide groups were similar.

Similarly, Chen et al[25] randomly assigned 193 patients to receive either carbon dioxide or air insufflation during insertion when colonoscopy was performed. All patients had carbon dioxide during withdrawal of the colonoscope. The mean pain scores during intubation in both groups were low (2 to 3 on a 10-point visual analog scale [VAS]), and the mean pain score at 1, 3, 6, and 24 hours after colonoscopy was 0 in both groups. Thus, carbon dioxide insufflation during withdrawal rather than insertion may be the most important factor for reducing postprocedure pain.

The removal of large colonic lesions typically requires longer procedure times and more air insufflation, thus potentially increasing the incidence of pain. Bassan et al[26] studied 524 consecutive patients undergoing endoscopic resection of sessile colorectal polyps 20 mm or larger. A total of 334 patients received air insufflation, whereas 190 patients had procedures performed with carbon dioxide. Carbon dioxide use was associated with an 82% reduction in postpolypectomy admissions because of severe pain, from 5.7% to 1.0% ($P = .006$). This led to an overall 62% reduction in the postpolypectomy admission rate from 8.9% to 3.4% ($P = .01$).

In an analogous study of potentially difficult colonoscopies performed by less-experienced endoscopists, the mean VAS pain scores were better in the patients who received carbon dioxide insufflation ($n = 30$) than in those who received air insufflation ($n = 31$).[27]

Endoscopic submucosal dissection (ESD) is another technique for resecting large colonic polyps. ESD can be time consuming, and standard air insufflation may potentially result in severe pain when compared with traditional screening colonoscopies.

In a pilot study by Saito et al,[28] 35 patients had ESD with carbon dioxide insufflation throughout the procedure while under conscious sedation. They were compared with a historic control group of 35 patients who received air insufflation during their colonic ESD procedure. The mean procedure time was 90 ± 57 minutes in the carbon dioxide–insufflation group and 100 ± 80 minutes in the air-insufflation group ($P =$ NS). Two patients in the carbon dioxide–insufflation group complained of mild abdominal discomfort during the procedure, and none reported pain 1 hour postprocedure. Although the historic control group that received air was not evaluated for abdominal pain, there was a significant increase in the dose of midazolam needed for sedation in the carbon dioxide–insufflation group (9.7 ± 5.9 mg as compared with 5.6 ± 4.9 mg; $P = 0.005$).

In a recent meta-analysis by Wang et al[29] of 13 randomized, controlled trials of colonoscopy with air vs carbon dioxide, there was an overall reduced postprocedure pain intensity with carbon dioxide insufflation. More patients in the carbon dioxide–insufflation group were pain free at 1 hour (relative risk, 1.84; 95% confidence interval, 1.37 to 2.47) and 6 hours (relative risk, 1.28; 95% confidence interval, 1.14 to 1.44) after colonoscopy.

Although many studies have supported the reduction of pain observed after colonoscopy with carbon dioxide insufflation, few studies have investigated the effects on pain during the procedure. In a recent intention-to-treat analysis by Amato et al,[30] 115 patients having colonoscopy with carbon dioxide requested less sedation, on average, than the 113 patients in the air-insufflation group ($P = .04$), suggesting that they experienced less pain during their procedures.

Because carbon dioxide is absorbed rapidly from the colon into the plasma, there is some concern regarding an effect on respiration. In a systematic review by Dellon et al,[31] nine randomized, controlled trials comparing carbon dioxide and air insufflation for colonoscopies (6), flexible sigmoidoscopy (1), endoscopic retrograde cholangiopancreatography (1), and double balloon enteroscopy (1) were identified. There were no adverse pulmonary events in any study.

Conclusion

Carbon dioxide and water are viable alternatives to air insufflation during colonoscopy. Their primary benefit appears to be reducing pain during and after the procedure, which translates into increased patient comfort and may reduce the rate of postprocedure admissions and emergency room visits. Unlike the use of air and water, carbon dioxide typically involves additional hardware and expense. Carbon dioxide may be riskier for patients with carbon dioxide retention at baseline.[32] To date, there have been no head-to-head comparisons of carbon dioxide and water insufflation during colonoscopy, although such studies would be valuable. Similarly, the influence of alternative insufflation modalities on polyp and adenoma detection rates needs to be further studied.

References

1. Denberg TD, Melhado TV, Coombes JM, et al. Predictors of nonadherence to screening colonoscopy. *J Gen Intern Med.* 2005;20(11):989-995.
2. Cooper GS, Kou TD, Rex DK. Complications following colonoscopy with anesthesia assistance: a population-based analysis. *JAMA Intern Med.* 2013;173(7):551-556.
3. Pohl J, Messer I, Behrens A, Kaiser G, Mayer G, Ell C. Water infusion for cecal intubation increases patient tolerance, but does not improve intubation of unsedated colonoscopies. *Clin Gastroenterol Hepatol.* 2011;9(12):1039-1043.e1.
4. Baumann UA. Water intubation of the sigmoid colon: water instillation speeds up left-sided colonoscopy. *Endoscopy.* 1999;31(4):314-317.
5. Hamamoto N, Nakanishi Y, Morimoto N, et al. A new water instillation method for colonoscopy without sedation as performed by endoscopists-in-training. *Gastrointest Endosc.* 2002;56(6):825-828.

6. Leung FW. Water exchange may be superior to water immersion for colonoscopy. *Clin Gastroenterol Hepatol.* 2011;9(12):1012-1014.
7. Leung JW, Mann S, Leung FW. Options for screening colonoscopy without sedation: a pilot study in United States veterans. *Aliment Pharmacol Ther.* 2007;26(4):627-631.
8. Leung FW, Amato A, Ell C, et al. Water-aided colonoscopy: a systematic review. *Gastrointest Endosc.* 2012;76(3):657-666.
9. Lee BY, Katon R, Herzig D, Fennerty MB. Warm water infusion during sedated colonoscopy does not decrease amount of sedation medication used. *Gastrointest Endosc.* 2012;76(6):1182-1187.
10. Leung FW. Is there a place for sedationless colonoscopy? *J Interv Gastroenterol.* 2011;1(1):19-22.
11. Ramirez FC, Leung FW. The water method for aiding colonoscope insertion: the learning curve of an experienced colonoscopist. *J Interv Gastroenterol.* 2011;1(3):97-101.
12. Lin S, Zhu W, Xiao K, et al. Water intubation method can reduce patients' pain and sedation rate in colonoscopy: a meta-analysis. *Dig Endosc.* 2013;25(3):231-240.
13. Rabenstein T, Radaelli F, Zolk O. Warm water infusion colonoscopy: a review and meta-analysis. *Endoscopy.* 2012;44(10):940-951.
14. Vemulapalli KC, Rex DK. Water immersion simplifies cecal intubation in patients with redundant colons and previous incomplete colonoscopies. *Gastrointest Endosc.* 2012;76(4):812-817.
15. Bourke MJ, Rex DK. Tips for better colonoscopy from two experts. *Am J Gastroenterol.* 2012;107(10): 1467-1472.
16. Luo H, Zhang L, Liu X, et al. Water exchange enhanced cecal intubation in potentially difficult colonoscopy. Unsedated patients with prior abdominal or pelvic surgery: a prospective, randomized, controlled trial. *Gastrointest Endosc.* 2013;77(5):767-773.
17. Cammarota G, Cesaro P, Cazzato A, et al. The water immersion technique is easy to learn for routine use during EGD for duodenal villous evaluation: a single-center 2-year experience. *J Clin Gastroenterol.* 2009;43(3):244-248.
18. Binmoeller KF, Weilert F, Shah J, Bhat Y, Kane S. "Underwater" EMR without submucosal injection for large sessile colorectal polyps (with video). *Gastrointest Endosc.* 2012;75(5):1086-1091.
19. Frossard J-L, Gervaz P, Huber O. Water-immersion sigmoidoscopy to treat acute GI bleeding in the perioperative period after surgical colorectal anastomosis. *Gastrointest Endosc.* 2010;71(1):167-170.
20. Brandt LJ, Boley SJ, Sammartano R. Carbon dioxide and room air insufflation of the colon: effects on colonic blood flow and intraluminal pressure in the dog. *Gastrointest Endosc.* 1986;32(5):324-329.
21. Bretthauer M, Hoff GS, Thiis-Evensen E, Huppertz-Hauss G, Skovlund E. Air and carbon dioxide volumes insufflated during colonoscopy. *Gastrointest Endosc.* 2003;58(2):203-206.
22. Stevenson GW, Wilson JA, Wilkinson J, Norman G, Goodacre RL. Pain following colonoscopy: elimination with carbon dioxide. *Gastrointest Endosc.* 1992;38(5):564-567.
23. Sumanac K, Zealley I, Fox BM, et al. Minimizing postcolonoscopy abdominal pain by using CO(2) insufflation: a prospective, randomized, double blind, controlled trial evaluating a new commercially available CO(2) delivery system. *Gastrointest Endosc.* 2002;56(2):190-194.
24. Hsu W-H, Sun M-S, Lo H-W, Tsai C-Y, Tsai Y-J. Carbon dioxide insufflation during withdrawal of the colonoscope improved postprocedure discomfort: a prospective, randomized, controlled trial. *Kaohsiung J Med Sci.* 2012;28(5):265-269.
25. Chen PJ, Li CH, Huang TY, et al. Carbon dioxide insufflation does not reduce pain scores during colonoscope insertion in unsedated patients: a randomized, controlled trial. *Gastrointest Endosc.* 2013;77(1):79-89.
26. Bassan MS, Holt B, Moss A, Williams SJ, Sonson R, Bourke MJ. Carbon dioxide insufflation reduces number of postprocedure admissions after endoscopic resection of large colonic lesions: a prospective cohort study. *Gastrointest Endosc.* 2013;77(1):90-95.
27. Uraoka T, Kato J, Kuriyama M, et al. CO(2) insufflation for potentially difficult colonoscopies: efficacy when used by less experienced colonoscopists. *World J Gastroenterol.* 2009;15(41):5186-5192.
28. Saito Y, Uraoka T, Matsuda T, et al. A pilot study to assess the safety and efficacy of carbon dioxide insufflation during colorectal endoscopic submucosal dissection with the patient under conscious sedation. *Gastrointest Endosc.* 2007;65(3):537-542.
29. Wang WL, Wu ZH, Sun Q, et al. Meta-analysis: the use of carbon dioxide insufflation vs. room air insufflation for gastrointestinal endoscopy. *Aliment Pharmacol Ther.* 2012;35(10):1145-1154.
30. Amato A, Radaelli F, Paggi S, Baccarin A, Spinzi G, Terruzzi V. Carbon dioxide insufflation or warm-water infusion versus standard air insufflation for unsedated colonoscopy: a randomized controlled trial. *Dis Colon Rectum.* 2013;56(4):511-518.

31. Dellon ES, Hawk JS, Grimm IS, Shaheen NJ. The use of carbon dioxide for insufflation during GI endoscopy: a systematic review. *Gastrointest Endosc.* 2009;69(4):843-849.
32. Chao I-F, Chiu H-M, Liu W-C, Liu C-C, Wang H-P, Cheng Y-J. Significant hypercapnia either in CO(2)-insufflated or air-insufflated colonoscopy under deep sedation. *Acta Anaesthesiol Taiwan.* 2010;48(4):163-166.

Please visit www.routledge.com/9781617116148 to access additional material.

4

External Pressure During Colonoscopy
How and When to Use It

Nicolas Villa, MD and Waqar Qureshi, MD, FRCP

The incidence and mortality of colorectal cancer in the United States have decreased during recent years in part because of an awareness of risk factors, the widespread availability of screening colonoscopy, and improved treatment options.[1] It has also been attributed to increased detection and removal of precancerous polyps as a result of colorectal cancer screening.[2-4]

The quality of colonoscopic examinations has come under particular scrutiny, with the current literature emphasizing the need for a high-quality examination to increase the detection and removal of adenomatous polyps and reduce the risk of colorectal cancer overall. The quality of bowel cleansing, colonoscopic withdrawal time, and adenoma detection rates are some of the quality measures being studied.

The United States Multi-Society Task Force in Colorectal Cancer recommends that colonoscopists be able to achieve cecal intubation in 90% of all cases and 95% of screening colonoscopies.[5] Occasionally, the colonoscopist is faced with a difficult colon, defined as one in which the endoscopist encounters difficulties in reaching the cecum with the colonoscope.[6]

The single most important factor that determines the success of colonoscopy is the endoscopist's experience, although even the most experienced endoscopist may struggle in certain situations because colonoscopy can be a technically challenging procedure. Such challenges are encountered more commonly in patients with a suboptimal bowel preparation, severe diverticulosis, tortuous colons, an obese body habitus, a history of previous abdominal or pelvic surgeries, and the formation of colonoscopic loops, as well as in female and young patients. Any and all of these difficulties may cause a substantial increase in procedure length and may ultimately prevent cecal intubation.[6-9]

Adler DG, ed.
Core Concepts in Colonoscopy (pp 39-50).

Several techniques have been used to offset these problems and make colonoscopy easier: water immersion, minimizing air insufflation or using carbon dioxide for bowel insufflation, using thinner endoscopes or variable-stiffness colonoscopes, fluoroscopy, changes in patient body position, loop reduction, and external compression.

This chapter will focus on the techniques of external compression of the abdomen as practiced during colonoscopy. These techniques often make the examination easier, limit patient discomfort, shorten examination time, and (in certain circumstances) may be the only way to reach the cecum or terminal ileum.[10]

Concept of External Compression During Colonoscopy

The primary goal of the external compression technique is to externally support (splint) the colonoscope and prevent looping. An experienced assistant who understands the principles of external compression can make the difference between success and failure. In addition, effective abdominal pressure may help prevent perforation by keeping the colon from stretching excessively as the assistant helps straighten the scope. Therefore, external compression makes colonoscopy safer and faster overall.

Before applying external pressure, one needs to have an idea of where the colonoscope is located anatomically within the colon and what sort of loop might be present. Although this may sound simple, in reality the endoscopist can only make an educated guess regarding the location of the tip of the endoscope and which type of loop may (or may not) be present. Nonetheless, with experience and time, many endoscopists can learn to accurately make these types of assessments. Knowing when to ask for external compression, and how it should be applied, is often critical to overall procedural success.

Some simple tricks and general rules of thumb can assist the endoscopist in judging the location of the colonoscope tip. This information is vital when external pressure is applied because it gives the assistant information about where external pressure is most likely to be effective.

The anal canal is approximately 3 cm long and extends to the squamocolumnar junction, or *dentate line*. The rectum measures 12 to 15 cm from the anal verge and contains the semilunar folds, or *valves of Houston*.

Beyond the rectum lies the sigmoid colon. The sigmoid colon can reach 40 to 70 cm or more in length when stretched by the colonoscope during insertion, but it typically extends to 30 to 35 cm beyond the rectum when the colonoscope is fully straightened. The sigmoid colon has a more tubular appearance because of its significantly thicker circular musculature. Vascular pulsations of the adjacent left iliac artery are often visible in the sigmoid colon, providing another clue to the endoscopist about his or her location during the examination.

Above the sigmoid colon lies the descending colon. The descending colon is relatively straight and can be as long as 20 cm. This segment is usually traversed quickly because its position is fixed by its location within the retroperitoneum.

Above the descending colon is the splenic flexure. This is an area of fixed angulation in the colon. The mucosa at the splenic flexure often has a blue-gray discoloration caused by the adjacent spleen.

After the endoscopist rounds the splenic flexure, the transverse colon is entered. Approximately 40 cm long, the transverse colon is notable for its triangular-shaped lumen due to wall tension by the 3 separate longitudinal ribbons of smooth muscle on the outside of the colon known as the *taenia coli*. Although the taenia coli are present around other segments of the colon, it is in the transverse colon that they make their presence felt most acutely. Marked aortic or cardiac pulsation may be seen in the transverse colon. The hepatic flexure, which lies just proximal to the transverse colon, is another point of fixed angulation that is identified easily by a blue-gray discoloration due to the adjacent liver. The mucosal discoloration at the hepatic flexure is usually much more prominent than that seen at the splenic flexure.

The 20-cm ascending colon, which is proximal to the hepatic flexure, is usually straight because it is fixed by the retroperitoneum. It is also thin walled and may have a triangular lumen. It is connected to the cecum, which is the beginning of the large intestine. In most patients, the cecum is approximately 5 cm long. Although one would think the sum of the lengths of these separate segments of the colon would provide its total length, in practice the cecum is often reached when 60 to 80 cm of the endoscope has been inserted after the shaft is straightened and all loops are reduced.[11]

External Compression Techniques and When to Use Them

At the beginning of the colonoscopy, the patient is placed in the left lateral position with his or her buttocks at the edge of the table. The patient's legs may be straight, bent, or a combination thereof (eg, bottom leg straight and top leg bent).

After a digital rectal examination is performed, the colonoscope is well lubricated and inserted into the patient's anus. The left hand is used to hold the colonoscope control head and the right hand holds the shaft of the endoscope 10 to 20 cm from the anus so that force is transmitted straight up through the endoscope in an attempt to minimize looping.

As a general rule, during insertion of the colonoscope, one should insufflate as little air as possible—just enough to see the lumen. As more air is insufflated, the bowel distends and lengthens. This increases patient discomfort and makes it more difficult to advance the colonoscope than it would be in a decompressed colon.

It is important to keep the colonoscope as straight as possible during the entire procedure to prevent excess looping. The endoscope is straightened by withdrawal (pulling back), especially after negotiating a turn.

When significant looping occurs, such that the colonoscope will not advance or seems to withdraw when the shaft is advanced into the colon, external compression is needed. At this time, one should withdraw with clockwise torque to straighten the colonoscope as much as possible in addition to using air suctioning until the walls just begin to collapse.[12] External compression by the assistant may then be started from the endoscopist's side of the table or at the opposite side with the assistant facing the patient.

As a general principle, if abdominal pressure is applied to one area of the abdomen and is not effective, persistence is unlikely to produce the desired result; it is often best to move on and try to apply abdominal pressure at another location with the patient in the same position. Conversely, if abdominal pressure is unsuccessful when applied to one area of the abdomen, pressure to the same location can be repeated after changing the patient's position (eg, moving the patient from the left lateral position to the supine position).[10]

Abdominal pressure can be applied by several methods, all of which can be helpful. One or 2 hands can be used, as can the forearm (often in combination with the hands). The assistant providing pressure may apply counterpressure to the patient's back and may need to stand on a stool to apply pressure from the correct angle. The endoscopist should be mindful of the fact that applying external pressure can be physically demanding; if the assistant becomes fatigued, the pressure can be relieved or a second assistant may need to help.

Recommendations for Pressure at Specific Areas of the Colon

Rectosigmoid Colon

This area of the colon has the valves of Houston, which are sharply angulated curves in the bowel wall. The sigmoid colon is not fixed within the abdomen, and as such can be moved by the effects of the endoscope, air insufflation, or both. As such, minimal air should be insufflated into the sigmoid colon to reduce the risk of forming a loop in the first place. Difficulties in advancing the endoscope through the sigmoid colon are commonly caused by inexperience, diverticulosis, or previous abdominal/pelvic surgery.

If a loop develops in the sigmoid colon and reducing the loop does not allow the endoscope to advance, applying abdominal pressure to the suprapubic area is usually enough to assist one in moving the endoscope through the sigmoid colon.

If this is unsuccessful, another technique that can be used is the sigmoid lift (Figure 4-1). With the patient positioned on his or her left side, the assistant places his or her left hand superior to the patient's left pelvic bone and subsequently places the right hand under the left hand, thus rolling the left forearm toward the abdomen. This helps straighten the sigmoid and splint the scope simultaneously, both of which promote forward endoscope motion.

Junction of Sigmoid and Descending Colon

If a loop starts forming at the junction of the sigmoid and descending colon, the colonoscope can be withdrawn to the level of the rectosigmoid junction to straighten the scope. Abdominal pressure can be applied to the left lower abdomen to splint the sigmoid colon and minimize the chance of loop formation (Figure 4-2).

If this simple maneuver does not work (it may not be successful in obese patients), another option is to place the patient in a supine position and apply midabdominal pressure. This maneuver can fix the flexible sigmoid colon in the left lower abdomen. This maneuver can be enhanced further if the assistant's other hand is used on the patient's left lateral side to prevent movement of the sigmoid colon to the left side (Figure 4-3).

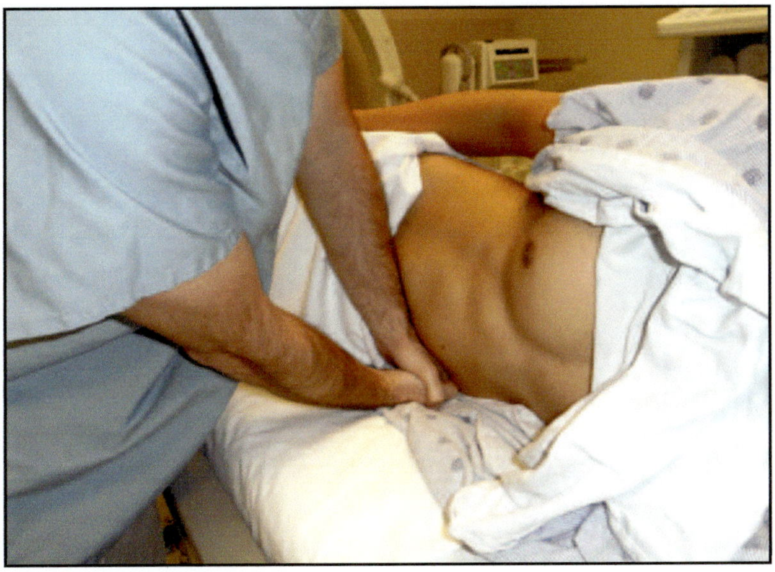

Figure 4-1. The sigmoid lift helps straighten the sigmoid and splint the scope to help it move forward.

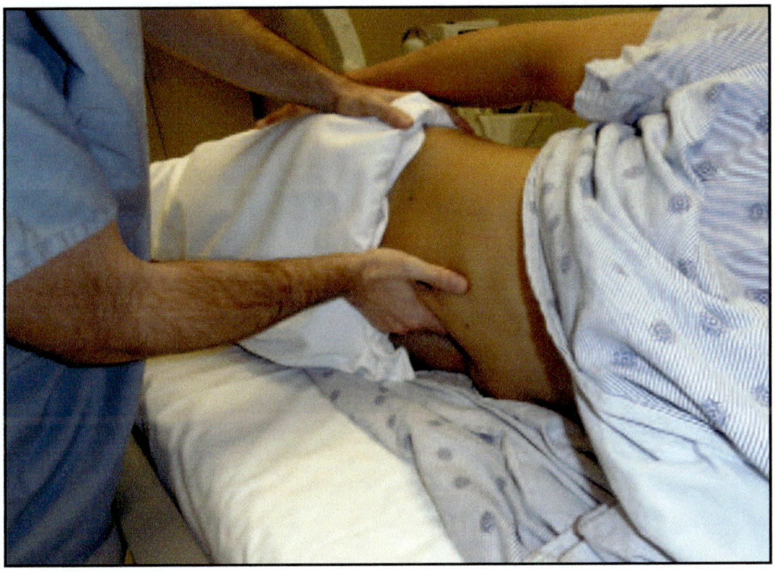

Figure 4-2. Pressure applied to the left lower abdomen to splint the sigmoid colon can prevent the formation of a loop.

Splenic Flexure

The splenic flexure is a fixed, angulated colonic structure that can sometimes be difficult to traverse. When one reaches this area, the colonoscope should be kept as straight as possible to minimize the risk of looping. If a loop forms and cannot be reduced (or if the loop reforms on repeated attempts to traverse the splenic flexure), abdominal pressure over the splenic flexure can be applied with the patient in either the left lateral or supine position (Figure 4-4). If this fails to produce results, then applying pressure over the suprapubic and left midabdominal area with the patient in either the left lateral position or supine is the next option (Figure 4-5). This last maneuver can splint the rectosigmoid colon and the descending colon simultaneously to prevent loop formation.

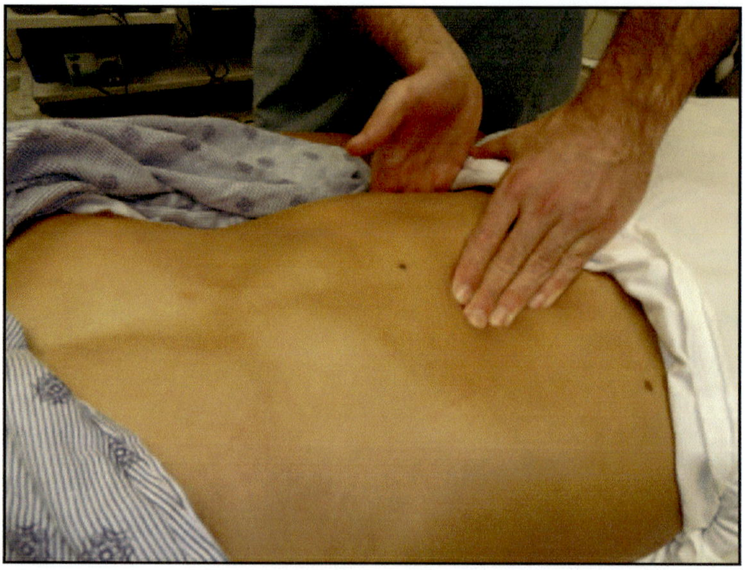

Figure 4-3. As a modification of the technique shown in Figure 4-2, pressure can be applied with the right hand to hold the sigmoid colon in place, which is especially useful in overweight patients.

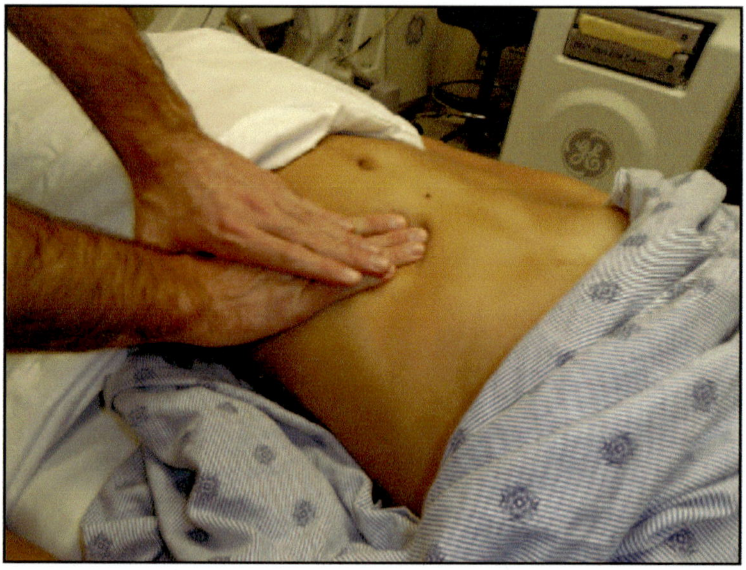

Figure 4-4. External pressure can be applied over the splenic flexure with the patient in the left lateral position or supine position to facilitate advancement of the colonoscope through the splenic flexure.

Transverse Colon

The transverse colon is a relatively floppy portion of the colon that is not adhered to the retroperitoneum and can descend into the pelvis and cause difficulties when the operator is advancing the colonoscope. Looping, with associated paradoxical motion (apparent retrograde motion of the endoscope when forward motion is applied as a result of looping), is common here. Pain also can occur if a loop forms. It is important to try to reduce as much as possible when traversing the transverse colon. Judicious use of suction with simultaneous clockwise rotation of the endoscope shaft on reaching the hepatic flexure can further minimize the risk of loop formation. These maneuvers can also be performed in the midtransverse colon prophylactically to avoid looping and falling back to the splenic flexure (with the resulting need to renegotiate this segment of the colon).

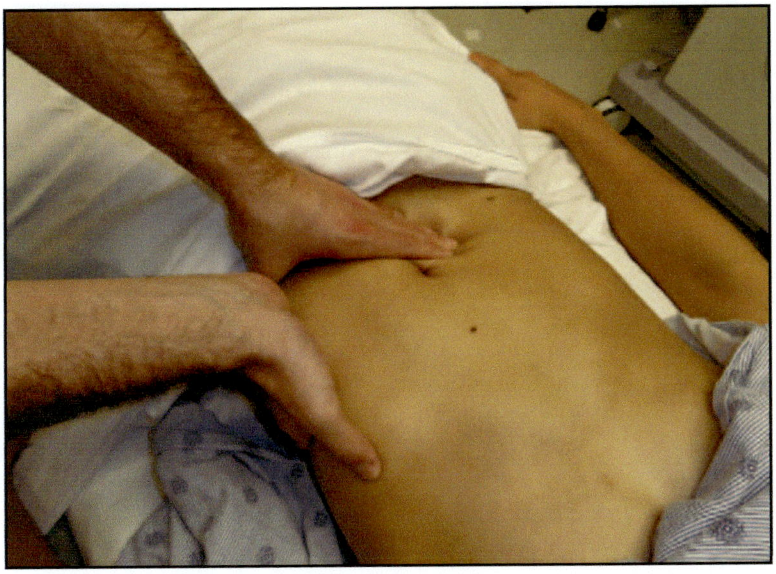

Figure 4-5. Applying pressure over the suprapubic and left midabdominal area with the patient in either the left lateral position or supine position can help the endoscopist advance beyond the splenic flexure in difficult cases.

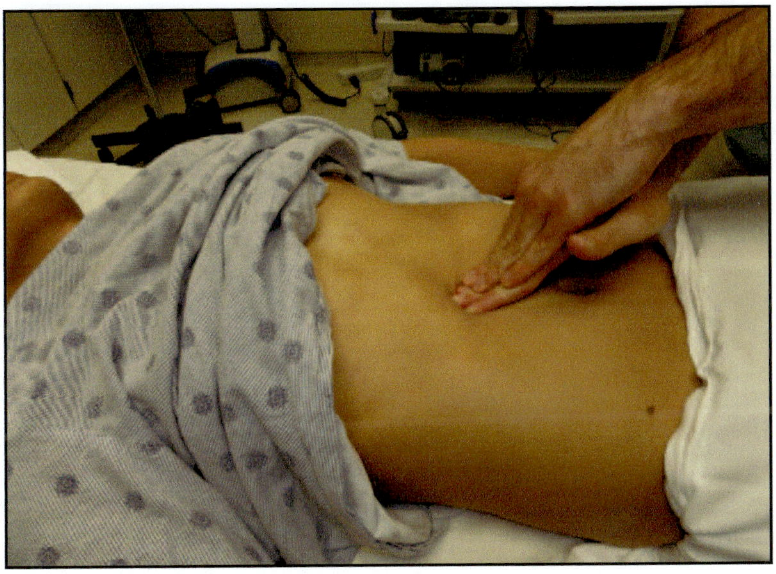

Figure 4-6. Difficulty in advancing the colonoscope through the transverse colon is overcome by applying pressure in a cranial direction above the umbilicus. This will straighten the transverse colon and simplify advancement of the colonoscope.

When one is having problems traversing the transverse colon, it is often helpful to place the patient in the supine position before applying abdominal pressure. The assistant can then try placing a hand (or hands) above the umbilicus and applying pressure toward the cranium. This can brace the transverse colon and minimize the risk of it descending into the lower abdomen, thus straightening the transverse colon and simplifying advancement of the colonoscope to the hepatic flexure (Figure 4-6).

Hepatic Flexure

Similar to the splenic flexure, the hepatic flexure is a fixed and angulated structure. If difficulties arise in transiting this point, and if endoscope reduction maneuvers and suctioning have been tried and failed, abdominal pressure is usually required. When one

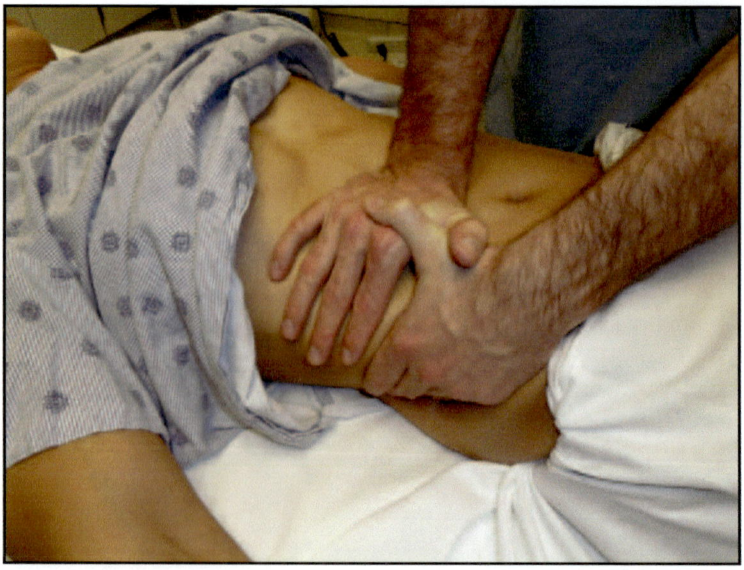

Figure 4-7. External pressure can be applied to the right flank over the hepatic flexure, making it easier to turn the endoscope tip through the hepatic flexure.

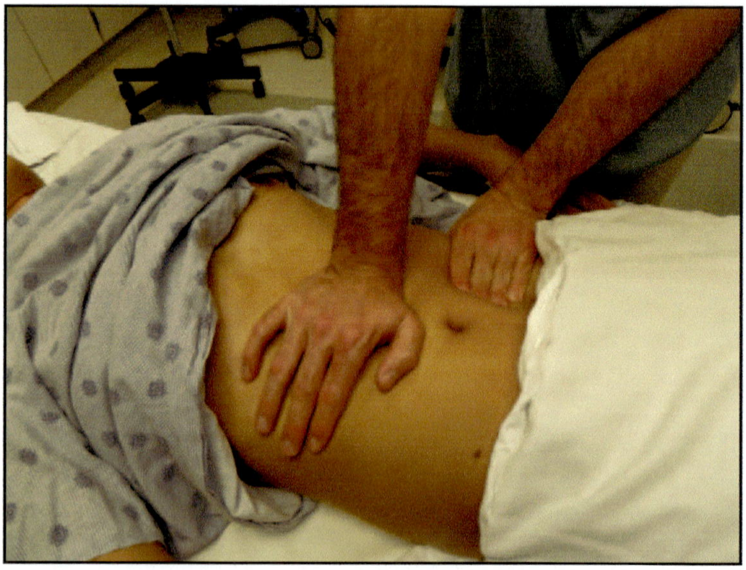

Figure 4-8. Pressure in the upper midabdomen (transverse area) and left lower quadrant (sigmoid area) also will help the endoscopist advance the colonoscope through the hepatic flexure.

is traversing the hepatic flexure, the patient can be placed supine and external pressure can be applied to the right flank over the hepatic flexure. This usually makes it easier for one to turn the endoscope tip through the hepatic flexure (Figure 4-7). If this does not help, the next option is to apply pressure in the upper midabdomen (transverse area) and left lower quadrant (sigmoid area) to brace the colon and endoscope at several locations at once (Figure 4-8).

Ascending Colon

In most patients, the ascending colon is easily traversed. If difficulties arise, often the most effective solution is simply to apply suction and collapse the ascending colon (functionally shortening the length of the colon). Air or carbon dioxide gas insufflated earlier in

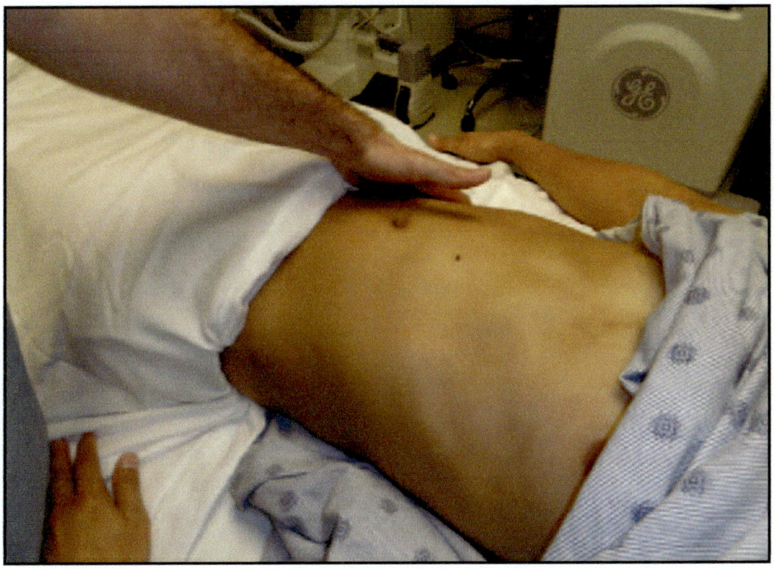

Figure 4-9. If the colonoscope will not enter the cecum, application of external pressure over the cecum (cecal lift) will facilitate the process (especially in a mobile cecum) and help when intubating the ileum.

the procedure tends to become trapped in the proximal colon, so experienced endoscopists will often reflexively apply suction immediately on entering the transverse colon. If a loop forms at this point, external pressure applied to the left flank or upper middle abdomen (or both simultaneously) can brace the endoscope and allow advancement to the cecum.

Cecum

A common difficulty encountered in the proximal colon is successful visualization of the ileocecal valve and cecum without easy access to the inside of the cecum itself. Remember, at this point the endoscope has been advanced to the proximal colon, and the endoscopist may observe a loss in 1-to-1 motion (signifying loop formation) and a decrease in overall mechanical effectiveness of the endoscope. In some circumstances, the endoscopist can simply push through the loop and "pop" into the cecum. If this is not successful, sometimes simply rolling the patient onto his or her back results in an effortless advancement into the cecum.

If abdominal pressure is required, this can be applied by several means. Applying external posterior-to-anterior pressure at the level of the cecum (the *cecal lift*) can be effective (especially in a mobile cecum). This maneuver also can be used to assist in accessing the terminal ileum in some patients after the cecum itself has been reached (Figure 4-9).

If the cecal lift does not help, 2-point pressure can be attempted (ie, pressure at the right upper quadrant and along the right flank simultaneously). Rarely, a 4-hand technique may be needed to reach the cecum, effectively bracing the entire endoscope to allow final advancement into the cecum (Figure 4-10). This technique requires 2 assistants. One person applies 2-handed pressure covering the sigmoid, splenic flexure, and transverse colon, while the other applies pressure covering the hepatic flexure and ascending colon. This maneuver, while rarely needed in practice, may be of great value in difficult cases.

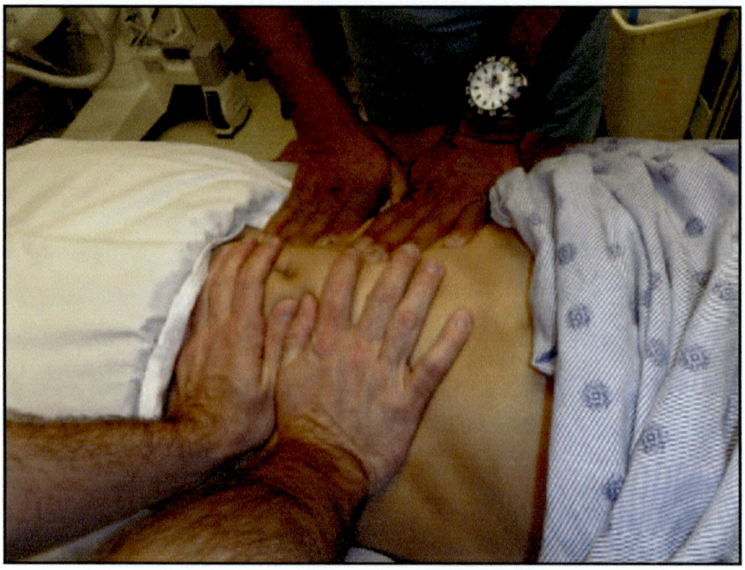

Figure 4-10. In difficult cases, the 4-hand technique may be necessary to reach the cecum.

Special Situations

At any point during the colonoscopy, if persistent looping occurs and external abdominal pressure with the patient in either the left lateral or supine position fails to remedy the problem, the patient can be rolled to the prone position. This maneuver may be especially helpful in obese patients. The obese patient's body weight can provide the equivalent of abdominal pressure over the entire abdominal wall. Additional abdominal pressure can be applied to the lateral aspects of the abdomen as well.

If the patient is in the left lateral position and abdominal pressure is required, it is often helpful for the assistant to stand behind the patient and reach over the abdomen while applying pressure in an anterior-to-posterior manner (a technique known as *Redwood pressure* for the clinic where it was developed). This technique allows the assistant to brace the entire patient with his or her body while applying pressure to maximize benefit, and it can be used for pressure anywhere in the abdomen.

On occasion, the open-hand pressure technique can cause wrist injury to the assistant, especially when the patient is in the left lateral position. Hyperextension of the wrist is the most common route to injury. Some authors advocate using the forearms (rather than hands) to apply pressure, but this may not be possible in all situations.[13,14] This technique is called the *forearm lift*. When using the forearm lift, the assistant places his or her left hand under the patient, extending his or her fingers or rolling them under to the knuckles. The wrist should be where the mattress and patient meet. Using the right hand, the assistant should pull the patient onto his or her left hand and onto the left forearm (Figure 4-11). This provides pressure to the sigmoid and lower abdomen along the midline. If additional pressure to the splenic flexure and/or transverse colon is desired, the assistant can place his or her right hand next to the left hand in the same fashion while the nurse provides counterpressure to the patient's back (Figure 4-12). This maneuver helps the assistant hold the pressure longer.

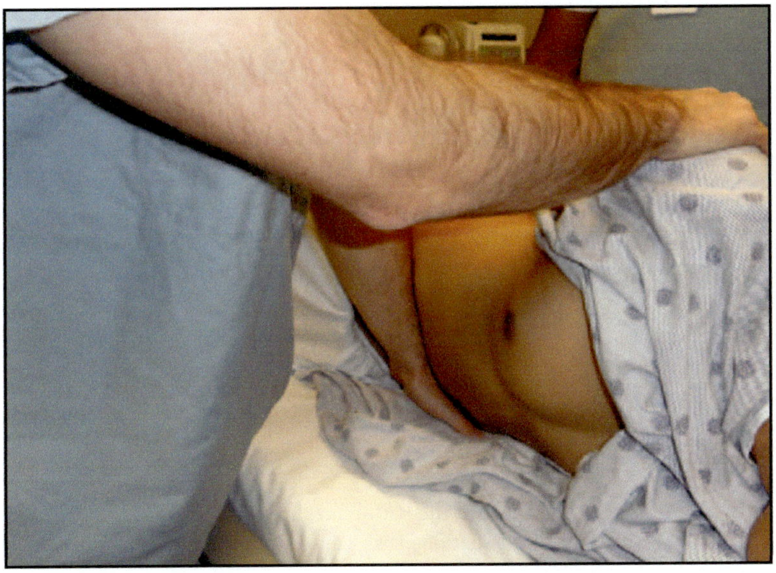

Figure 4-11. In the forearm lift, the assistant should place his or her left hand under the patient's left lower quadrant, extending the fingers or rolling them under to the knuckles. The wrist should be where the mattress and patient meet. Using the right hand, the assistant should pull the patient onto his or her left hand and onto the left forearm. This helps splint the sigmoid colon.

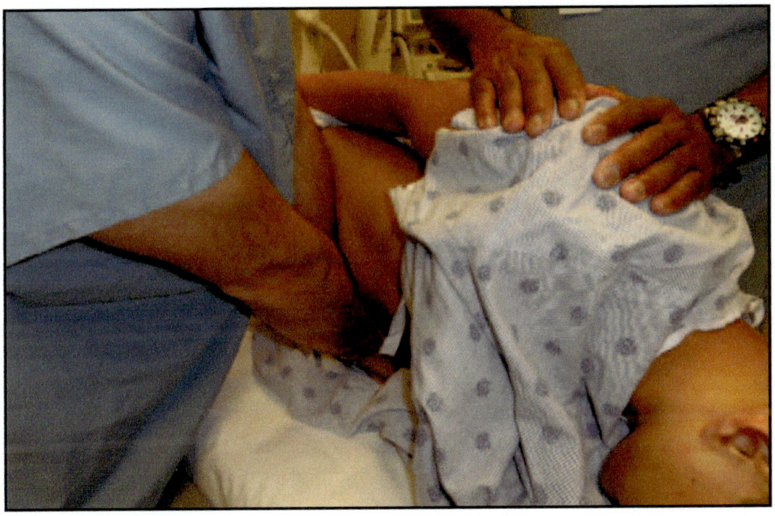

Figure 4-12. As a variation of the technique shown in Figure 4-11, the assistant can roll the patient gently forward.

In most cases, when pressure is applied with good body mechanics and positioning, it should be required for no longer than 20 to 30 seconds for each area of difficulty. If longer pressure application is expected, the assistant should be allowed to rest periodically, or a second assistant should be brought in to help.

Several key factors should be kept in mind when applying abdominal pressure during colonoscopy: (1) the assistant should be aware of the amount of pressure exerted to avoid injury to him- or herself or the patient; (2) the forearm technique is less likely to result in injury to the assistant compared with the open-hand technique; and (3) good body mechanics and positioning should be used for optimal comfort for the assistant and endoscopist.

Conclusion

Good endoscopic techniques combined with an understanding of the principles of external compression make colonoscopy safer and more efficient. The application of external abdominal pressure during a colonoscopy is an inexpensive, safe, and effective method to achieve cecal intubation in situations where endoscope advancement is difficult.

Good communication between the endoscopist and assistant is vital to good outcomes. Experience plays a key role in the successful application of external abdominal pressure, and experienced assistants should be asked to teach less-experienced assistants and physicians how and when external abdominal pressure should be applied.

References

1. Edwards BK, Ward E, Kohler BA, et al. Annual report to the nation on the status of cancer, 1975-2006, featuring colorectal cancer trends and impact of interventions (risk factors, screening, and treatment) to reduce future rates. *Cancer.* 2010;116(3):544-573.
2. Winawer SJ, Zauber AG, Ho MN, et al. Prevention of colorectal cancer by colonoscopic polypectomy. *N Engl J Med.* 1993;329:1977-1981.
3. Zauber AG, Winawer SJ, O'Brien MJ, et al. Colonoscopic polypectomy and long-term prevention of colorectal-cancer deaths. *N Engl J Med.* 2012;366:687-696.
4. American Cancer Society. *Colorectal Cancer Facts & Figures 2011-2013.* Atlanta, GA: American Cancer Society; 2011.
5. Rex D, Bond J, Winawer S, et al. Quality in the technical performance of colonoscopy and the continuous quality improvement process for colonoscopy: recommendations of the U.S. Multi-Society Task Force in Colorectal Cancer. *Am J Gastroenterol.* 2002;97:1296-1308.
6. Witte TN, Enns R. The difficult colonoscopy. *Can J Gastroenterol.* 2007;21(8):487-490.
7. Saunders BP, Fukumoto M, Hallingan S, et al. Why is colonoscopy more difficult in women? *Gastrointest Endosc.* 1996;43:124-126.
8. Anderson JC, Gonzales JD, Messina CR, et al. Factors that predict incomplete colonoscopy: thinner is not always better. *Am J Gastroenterol.* 2000;95:2784-2787.
9. Waye JD. Completing colonoscopy. *Am J Gastroenterol.* 2000;95:2681-2682.
10. Waye JD, Yessayan SA, Lewis BS, et al. The technique of abdominal pressure in total colonoscopy. *Gastrointest Endosc.* 1991;37:147-151.
11. Cotton PB, Williams CB. *Practical Gastrointestinal Endoscopy: The Fundamentals.* 6th ed. West Sussex, UK: Wiley-Blackwell; 2008:118-120.
12. Webb WA. Colonoscoping the "difficult colon." *Am Surg.* 1991;57:178-182.
13. Prechel JA, Young CJ, Hucke R, et al. The importance of abdominal pressure during colonoscopy: techniques to assist the physician and to minimize injury to the patient and assistant. *Gastroenterol Nurs.* 2005;28:232-236.
14. Prechel JA, Hucke R. Safe and effective abdominal pressure during colonoscopy: forearm versus open hand technique. *Gastroenterol Nurs.* 2009;32:27-30.

Please visit www.routledge.com/9781617116148 to access additional material.

5

Endoscopic Loops During Colonoscopy
How to Avoid Their Formation and How to Reduce Them When They Arise

Vivek Kaul, MD, FACG and Shivangi Kothari, MD

Colonoscopy is one of the most common endoscopic procedures in gastrointestinal endoscopy and an extremely effective tool for diagnostic and therapeutic maneuvers in the colon and rectum.[1] Given that the colon is a long, mobile, and flexible intra-abdominal organ with variable mesenteric attachments, passing a flexible endoscope from the rectum to the cecum can present a few challenges. One of the most common problems endoscopists face while performing colonoscopy is the formation of colonic/endoscopic loops, generally simply referred to as *loops*, which can be a source of discomfort or pain for the patient and prevent safe and efficient advancement of the colonoscope.[2] This chapter focuses on techniques that can help mitigate or prevent loop formation during colonoscopy and elaborates on some strategies that promote the resolution of loops when they do form.

Why Loops Form During Colonoscopy and the Types of Loops Encountered

Because of the flexible nature of the colon, its length, variable attachments to the mesentery, and its ability to distend (and simultaneously lengthen) with air insufflation, the path of a flexible colonoscope through the colon often assumes a nonlinear configuration, frequently resulting in loop formation. The loop consists of both the inserted instrument and the segment of colon that it is within.

Several distinct types of loops have been described, all of which essentially hinder instrument advancement and are invariably the cause of discomfort or pain during colonoscopy. In addition, if brute force (instead of proper technique) is used to counter this looping, iatrogenic injury (most commonly perforation) can occur during the procedure.[3]

Adler DG, ed.
Core Concepts in Colonoscopy (pp 51-60).

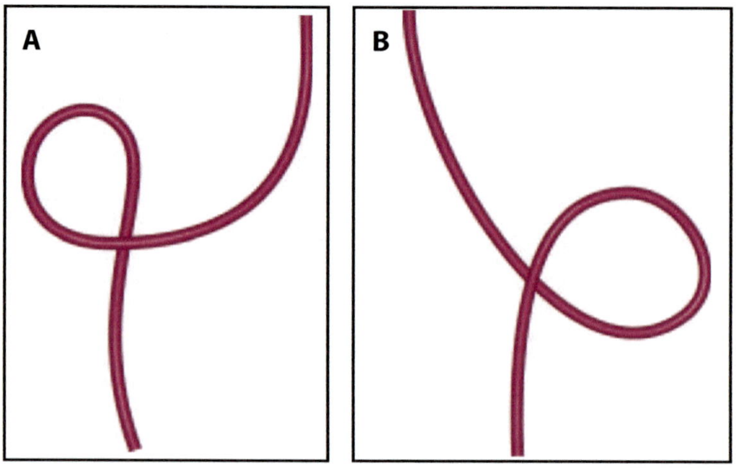

Figure 5-1. (A) The alpha loop. (B) Variation on the alpha loop reduced by the same maneuver.

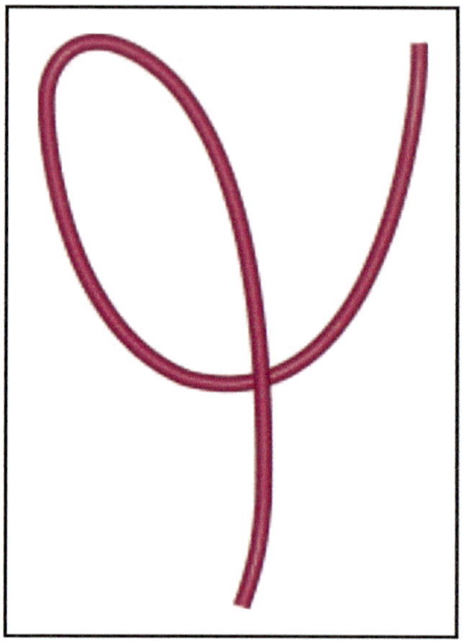

Figure 5-2. The reverse alpha loop.

The various types of endoscopic loops are depicted in Figures 5-1 through 5-5. The alpha, reverse alpha, and N loops typically form within the sigmoid and left colon segments. Alpha loops represent the formation of a complete spiral by the colonoscope and are right-handed loops (the spiral forms in a clockwise direction). Reverse alpha loops represent a left-handed or counterclockwise spiral. N loops roughly emulate the shape of the letter *n* when written in cursive and can apply pressure to the colon and mesentery at multiple points. The gamma loop is usually seen in a redundant transverse colon with a lax phrenicocolic ligament and results in an endoscopic loop that descends toward the pelvis. The deep transverse loop usually results from an anatomic variation at the splenic flexure, where the instrument passes laterally instead of medially around the flexure.

It should be stressed that loop formation is extremely common and not a sign of poor operator performance. All endoscopists encounter looping during colonoscopy, but experienced endoscopists take steps to minimize the risk of loop formation, recognize loop

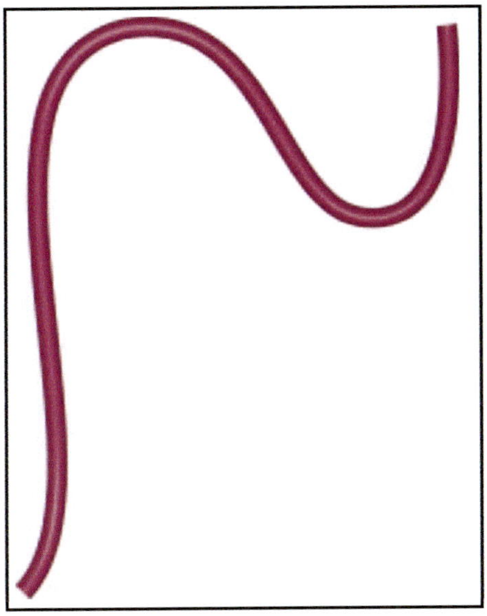

Figure 5-3. The N loop.

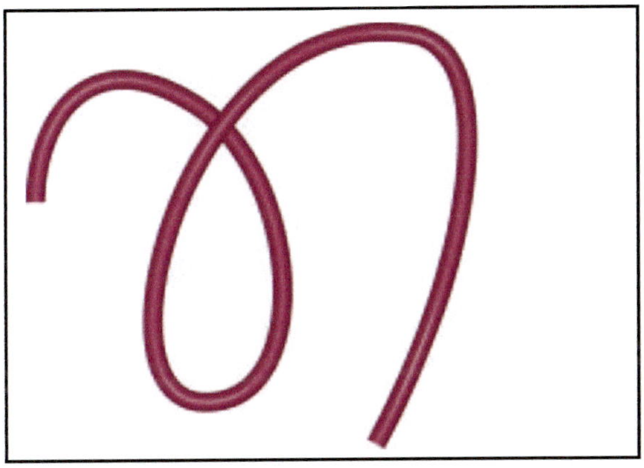

Figure 5-4. The gamma loop.

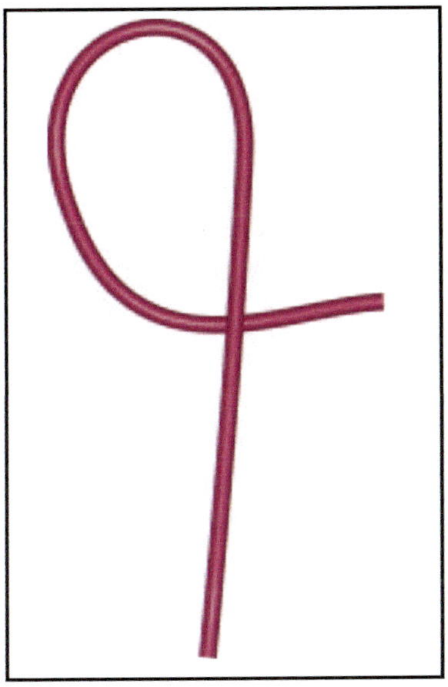

Figure 5-5. The deep transverse loop.

formation when it occurs, and reduce loops effectively to allow the procedure to proceed in a safe and timely manner.

Factors Affecting Endoscopic Loop Formation During Colonoscopy

The factors affecting formation of endoscopic loops during colonoscopy can be divided into patient-, instrument-, and endoscopist-related variables.[4] These factors are listed in Table 5-1.

- *Patient-related factors*: These primarily relate to alterations in colonic and/or pelvic anatomy in an individual patient. Any postsurgical (or postinflammatory) adhesions, a high degree of colonic fixity (whether due to disease or mesenteric attachments), and the length and degree of redundancy of the colon all affect the frequency of loop formation.
- *Instrument-related factors*: In general, the more flexible the endoscope, the greater the tendency to loop within the colon. Similarly, narrow-caliber endoscopes (pediatric colonoscopes) may be more prone to loop formation.
- *Endoscopist- and technique-related factors*: Variations in technique, operator experience, and abdominal pressure; changes in patient position; and the extent of air insufflation all affect loop formation during colonoscopy.

Minimizing or Avoiding Loop Formation During Colonoscope Insertion

The most important principle for avoiding loop formation during colonoscopy is to use proper technique during instrument insertion and advancement. Although some transient looping is inevitable given that both the colon and endoscope are flexible, every effort should be made to keep the instrument configuration as straight as possible throughout the examination to facilitate efficient and painless advancement to the cecum.

Before starting the procedure, one should check for any loops in the colonoscope outside the patient or in the umbilical cord. Once the colonoscope is inserted, one should avoid simply pushing in, especially when clear luminal views are not available, because this will likely result in early loop formation in the rectosigmoid and left colon. These alpha and N loops can be a source of significant pain for the patient and frustration for the endoscopist (see Figures 5-1 and 5-3).

Although it may seem counterintuitive during endoscope insertion, frequent, intermittent withdrawal and straightening or shortening of the instrument are key to eliminating loops as they form and maintaining the endoscope in a linear configuration. It is the mastery of this push-and-pull technique that distinguishes the expert colonoscopist from a novice.[5,6] Experienced endoscopists thus appear to be withdrawing the endoscope as much as they insert it on their way to the cecum.

Table 5-1. Factors Affecting Loop Formation

A. Patient related
- Colonic fixity vs redundancy
- Variability of mesenteric attachments
- Colonic length
- Pericolonic adhesions

B. Instrument related
- Flexible/small-caliber endoscope (more looping)
- Loops in endoscope outside patient (umbilicus)

C. Endoscopist/technique related
- Operator experience
- Operator technique (push/pull preferred)
- Degree of air or carbon dioxide insufflation
- Abdominal pressure
- Patient repositioning

Management and Resolution of Loops When They Form

Alpha Loop

This type of loop typically occurs in the sigmoid and descending colon, usually as a result of a long mesenteric attachment in the absence of adhesions. Alpha loops tend to form as one approaches the splenic flexure but can occur earlier in the procedure. If an alpha loop is formed, forward movement can become extremely limited. In this situation, the recommended strategy is to reduce the loop by applying simultaneous clockwise shaft rotation and withdrawing the instrument. This maneuver should be gentle and atraumatic as one monitors for any undue patient discomfort or resistance to endoscope withdrawal.

Attempts to reduce the loop too soon may result in the formation of an N loop, which is more difficult to manage, or repeated failure to maintain a stable position in the left colon.

Reverse Alpha Loop

If a sigmoid colon loop is formed and does not respond easily to the loop-reduction maneuver described previously, then one should suspect that a reverse alpha loop has formed. This type of loop typically occurs with a hypermobile left colon, allowing for an anticlockwise loop formation. Combined withdrawal and counterclockwise rotation are required to straighten the instrument and allow forward movement.

N (Spiral Sigmoid) Loop

This type of loop assumes a spiral 3-dimensional configuration, and, given its shape, any attempt to push the instrument forward stretches the sigmoid colon up toward the diaphragm, causing significant pain for the patient. Once the loop is recognized, reinsertion with external manual pressure on the sigmoid may reduce the size of the loop and allow instrument advancement. Another approach to N loops involves flexing the tip of the endoscope while withdrawing the endoscope with clockwise torque. The N loop tends to be more difficult to manage than the alpha loop. In addition, problems related to instrument advancement in the proximal colon are usually related to persistent N loop formation in the distal colon.

Gamma Loop

In patients with significant redundancy of the transverse colon, the endoscope may assume a gamma-loop orientation. Gamma loops are often a significant impediment to cecal intubation because they limit forward motion and may produce paradoxical motion. Once formed, this type of loop can be difficult to remove. Strong clockwise torque combined with simultaneous withdrawal of the endoscope may help eliminate the loop in some cases. Subsequent reinsertion combined with abdominal pressure may be helpful to avoid recurrent loop formation.

Deep Transverse Colon Loop

This results from anatomic variation at the splenic flexure where the endoscope passes laterally instead of medially around the flexure. Hooking the endoscope, withdrawing it, and then readvancing with abdominal pressure will reduce the risk of recurrent looping.

Transferring the Loop to the Umbilical Cord of the Endoscope

A helpful trick is to transfer a loop in the insertion tube to the umbilical cord of the endoscope. This involves completely rotating the entire endoscope and insertion tube together so they are straight while creating a loop in the umbilical cord behind the endoscopist (Figure 5-6). This results in a tremendous release of tension from the insertion tube. This may be difficult for novice endoscopists because the endoscope may fall back toward the rectum during the rotation, but once mastered, many find this an indispensable maneuver.

Colonoscopy Overview: Loop Formation and Reduction

Traversing the Rectum

In most patients, the rectum poses no obstacle for endoscope advancement. In some patients, most notably female patients with a history of low pelvic surgery, there may be severe angulation within the rectum itself that is difficult to traverse. External pressure

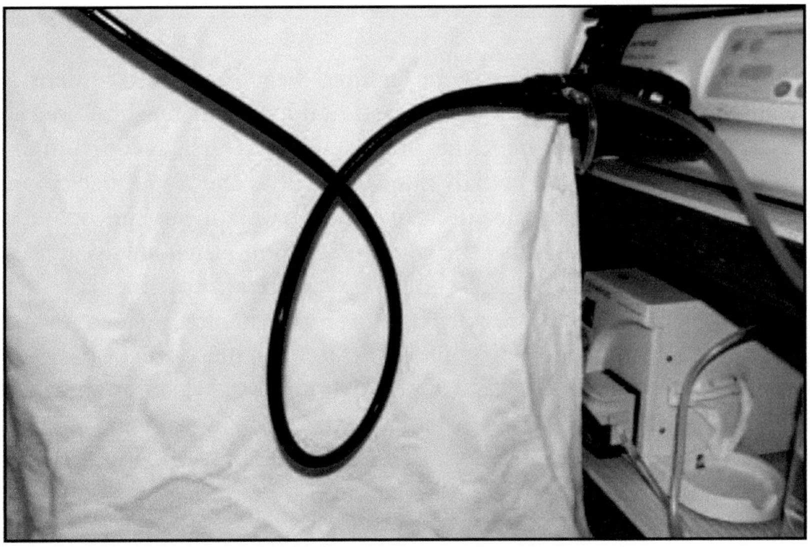

Figure 5-6. A loop in the insertion tube has been transferred to the umbilical cord.

may be of limited value when the endoscope tip is in the rectum, and switching from an adult colonoscope to a pediatric colonoscope is often the best strategy to try initially. Rarely, an upper endoscope is required to traverse a severe focal rectal angulation.

Traversing the Sigmoid and Descending Colon

The colonoscope should be held approximately 15 to 20 cm from the anus, with the endoscopist assuming a relaxed, comfortable stance at the bedside. Initial navigation through the sigmoid colon and the junction between the sigmoid and descending colon is often the most challenging part of the entire procedure. By applying appropriate colonoscope shaft torque (twisting force) along with up/down motions of the scope tip, one can "slalom" through the sharp angulations and turns in the rectosigmoid colon. Use of the lateral ratchet may help when negotiating tight turns. Using coordinated movements of the left thumb on the big (up/down) wheel and the right hand on the endoscope shaft, it is possible to pass the instrument through the sigmoid and left colon without creating any significant loops or discomfort for the patient.

Alpha-loop formation is common in the sigmoid colon. If an alpha loop does begin to form, clockwise rotation (torque) along with simultaneous and slight withdrawal of the instrument will usually straighten the configuration and allow more 1-to-1 motion within the colonic lumen.

Overangulation, created by using too much deflection of one or both wheels, usually results in a J-shaped configuration at the instrument tip. This is counterproductive to forward advancement and can result in additional loop formation when further advancement is attempted. Frequent endoscope withdrawal movement combined with suction and steering of the shaft will facilitate advancement of the endoscope through the descending colon to the splenic flexure. Optimal insertion to the splenic flexure requires approximately 50 to 55 cm of endoscope; the operator should have a relaxed hold on the instrument. Upon reaching the splenic flexure, often one can see the triangular luminal shape of the distal transverse colon in the distance.

Traversing the Splenic Flexure

The colon proximal to the splenic flexure can be entered best if the instrument is straightened maximally at this point and if there are no residual loops in the sigmoid and left colon. Simultaneous tip angulation to view the proximal (transverse colon) lumen, luminal suction, and endoscope advancement usually allow entry into the transverse colon. If one does not experience proper 1-to-1 advancement of the instrument (ie, endoscope is being pushed in, but the tip is not advancing into the transverse colon), then an alpha or N loop is likely forming in the distal colon. The loop should be reduced if possible. If recurrent loop formation is encountered, external pressure on the sigmoid colon by an assistant can often facilitate instrument advancement.[7] If this still does not help, then changing the patient position from left lateral decubitus to supine or right lateral decubitus should help advance the endoscope. An acutely angled splenic flexure may be opened up and made easier to traverse with the patient rotated to a different position. Position changes sometimes can be difficult when patients are deeply sedated or are obese.

Traversing the Transverse Colon

Continued luminal suction ensures a short colonic length as the endoscope moves through the transverse colon and approaches the hepatic flexure. As the operator traverses the transverse colon, loop formation can occur in the left colon or the transverse colon itself. Gamma loops often are formed in the transverse colon and frequently require a combination of reduction and external pressure. Intermittent clockwise torque, hooking the endoscope tip using the big wheel, and short-segment withdrawal (back-and-forth movements) may be needed to keep the instrument straight as it approaches the hepatic flexure.

Traversing the Hepatic Flexure

The hepatic flexure can sometimes be challenging to negotiate even with good technique. The turn itself can be sharply angulated, and at this point, a significant amount of the colonoscope has been inserted into the patient, reducing effective force transmission. If sigmoid and transverse colon loops exist, it may be impossible to traverse the hepatic flexure. Suction combined with tip deflection and gentle instrument advancement usually allows forward movement across the flexure. External pressure in the left upper quadrant (and occasionally in the right upper quadrant) and changing the patient to the supine or prone position may be required to allow entry into the right colon if difficulties are encountered.

Traversing the Ascending Colon and Cecum

The ascending colon tends to be fairly straight, and entry into this structure often affords a view of the ileocecal valve. This sight may prompt the endoscopist to simply attempt to push his or her way into the cecum. More often than not, pushing at this stage results in loop formation in the transverse colon and a paradoxical movement of the endoscope back toward the hepatic flexure. To avoid this phenomenon, a gentle withdrawal and straightening of the colonoscope shaft, combined with suction, will move the tip closer to the ileocecal valve and allow easy intubation of the cecum itself. If the endoscope reaches the valve but does not enter the cecum easily, a change in patient position to supine (sometimes with gentle abdominal pressure) frequently helps advance the instrument tip into the cecum.

An important caveat: it is difficult to intubate the ileocecal valve to evaluate the ileum if the endoscope is looped anywhere along its path. Hence, if ileal intubation is imperative, it is critical that the endoscope be as straight and relaxed as possible as it enters the cecum.

Additional Points to Consider

Although modifications in technique and specific maneuvers during the insertion phase are the mainstay for avoiding or eliminating colonoscopic looping, various other endoscope modifications and ancillary equipment have been evaluated over the years, with variable success reported in the literature. These include the Shapelock device (USGI Medical), which can fix the entire shape of the endoscope in any 3-dimensional configuration, variable-stiffness colonoscopes (as covered in Chapter 1), overtubes, and fluoroscopy and magnet-guided colonoscopy.[8-11] Variable-stiffness colonoscopes have become widely available and are quite popular among endoscopists. Many believe these devices can help minimize looping during colonoscopy and facilitate endoscope advancement, although the literature is equivocal regarding the definitive superiority of these devices over standard colonoscopes.[12]

Double balloon–assisted colonoscopy has emerged as an effective salvage tool, enabling total colonoscopy with a high degree of success in extremely tortuous and redundant colons where cecal intubation is not achievable (because of loops, sharp angulation, or adherent bowel) despite using optimal standard techniques.[13]

Although these additional devices are available, it should be stressed that in the vast majority of cases, proper technique and adherence to basic principles of colonoscopy are more than adequate to surmount any potential obstacles.

Conclusion

Colonoscopy provides an effective diagnostic and therapeutic platform for a wide range of colorectal diseases. Patient anxiety related to intraprocedural discomfort and iatrogenic injuries are well-known issues. Loop formation during colonoscopy is a common phenomenon and has the potential to cause significant pain, discomfort, and colonic injury if not recognized and corrected promptly.

Implementation of proper techniques during colonoscopy will help one avoid loop formation and make the examination more efficient for the endoscopist and more comfortable for the patient.

References

1. Rex DK, Petrini JL, Baron TH, et al. Quality indicators for colonoscopy. *Gastrointest Endosc.* 2006;63(suppl 4):S16-S28.
2. Raskin JB, Nord HJ, eds. *Colonoscopy: Principles and Techniques.* Tokyo, Japan: Igaku-Shoin; 1995.

3. Lohsiriwat V. Colonoscopic perforation: incidence, risk factors, management and outcome. *World J Gastroenterol.* 2010;16(4):425-430.
4. Cotton PB, Williams CB, eds. Colonoscopy and flexible sigmoidoscopy. In: *Practical Gastrointestinal Endoscopy.* 4th ed. London, UK: Blackwell Science; 1996:187-274.
5. Waye JD. Completing colonoscopy. *Am J Gastroenterol.* 2000;95:2681-2682.
6. Hunt RH, Waye JD. *Colonoscopy: Techniques, Clinical Practice and Colour Atlas.* London, UK: Chapman and Hall; 1981.
7. Waye JD, Yessayan SA, Lewis BS, Fabry TL. The technique of abdominal pressure in total colonoscopy. *Gastrointest Endosc.* 1991;37(2):147-151.
8. Hawari R, Pasricha PJ. Going for the loop: a unique overtube for the difficult colonoscopy. *J Clin Gastroenterol.* 2007;41(2):138-140.
9. Eickhoff A, Jakobs R, Kamal A, et al. In vitro evaluation of forces exerted by a new computer-assisted colonoscope (the Neo-Guide Endoscopy System). *Endoscopy.* 2006;38:1224-1229.
10. Raju GS, Rex DK, Kozarek RA, et al. A novel shape-locking guide for prevention of sigmoid looping during colonoscopy. *Gastrointest Endosc.* 2004;59:416-419.
11. Rex DK, Chen SC, Overhiser AJ. Colonoscopy technique in consecutive patients referred for prior incomplete colonoscopy. *Clin Gastroenterol Hepatol.* 2007;5:879-883.
12. Xie Q, Chen B, Liu L, Gan H. Does the variable stiffness colonoscope make colonoscopy easier? A meta-analysis. *BMC Gastroenterol.* 2012;12:151.
13. Pasha SF, Harrison ME, Das A, Corrado CM, Arnell KN, Leighton JA. Utility of double-balloon colonoscopy for completion of colon examination after incomplete colonoscopy with conventional colonoscope. *Gastrointest Endosc.* 2007;65:848-853.

6

Endoscopic Polypectomy Techniques

From Small to Large Lesions

Ali Siddiqui, MD; Serag Dredar, MD; Anna Strongin, MD; C. Andrew Kistler, MD, PharmD; and Shou-Jiang Tang, MD

Endoscopic polypectomy is one of the fundamental skills gastroenterologists develop throughout their careers. Although at times it may be considered a basic skill, it has made a substantial impact on the prevention of colorectal cancer (CRC), and in some cases, it is used to remove small primary CRCs.

Overall, the incidence and mortality rates for CRC have been declining in the United States during the past decade. Several factors have contributed to this decline, although appropriate CRC screening with colonoscopy and polypectomy has been reported to account for as much as 53% of the reduction in mortality.[1] As the benefits of CRC screening with colonoscopy continue to multiply, the technology and techniques used will expand. Basic and advanced polypectomy skills are being used more widely and are critical to endoscopic success in colonoscopy.

Forceps Polypectomy

Gastroenterologists frequently use forceps polypectomy to remove small or diminutive colon polyps. The advantages of this approach include the relative simplicity of the technique, minimal complication rate, widespread availability of the necessary equipment, and ease of tissue retrieval from the colon after the polypectomy.

Gastroenterologists have several different technique options when using forceps polypectomy, including different device sizes and the option of using electrocautery simultaneously. In addition, there are regular, large, and jumbo forceps. There are no guidelines that suggest one forceps over the other. It is important to note that several studies found that standard biopsy forceps leave behind residual polyp tissue more frequently than jumbo

Adler DG, ed.
Core Concepts in Colonoscopy (pp 61-80).

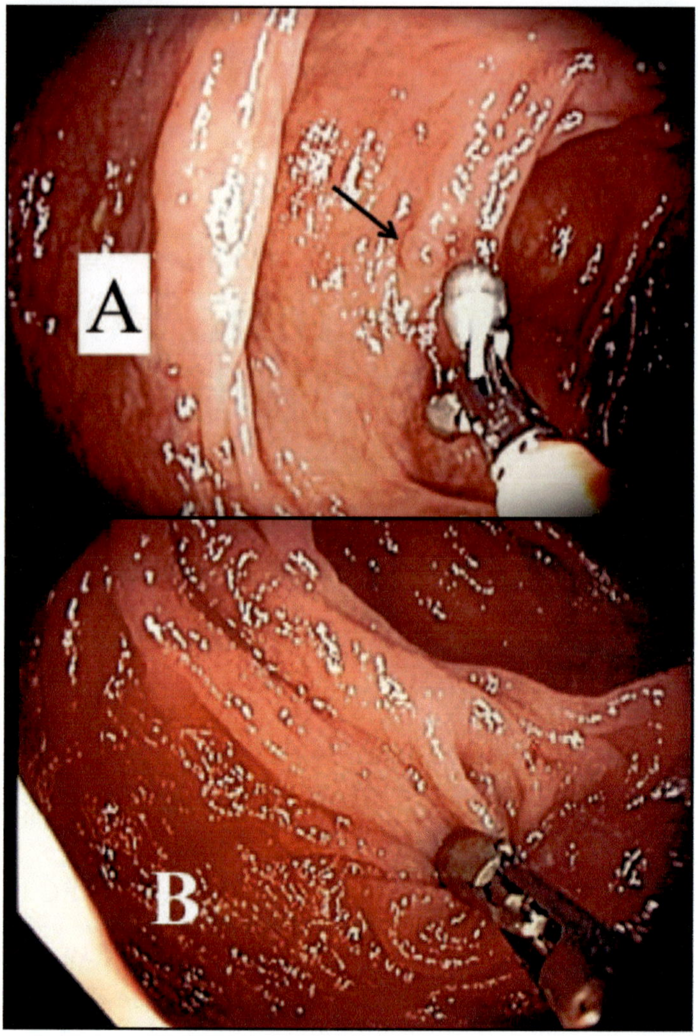

Figure 6-1. Small sessile polyps can be removed using cold forceps. Polyps that can be resected in a small number of bites are ideal for forceps resection. Estimation of polyp size can be aided by comparison to the size of the open forceps. (A) A small polyp about to be grasped in the open jaws of endoscopic forceps. (B) The polyp after it has been captured in the jaws of the forceps. (Reprinted with permission from Serag Dredar, MD.)

forceps.[2,3] However, the clinical implications of these findings are unclear because no studies have examined whether residual polyp tissue predicts a higher incidence of CRC down the line.

Forceps polypectomy without the use of electrocautery is known as a *cold forceps polypectomy*. With regard to technique, the polyp should be visualized in the 5- to 7-o'clock position for optimal accessibility. Subsequently, the forceps should be advanced through the working channel of the colonoscope, and the maximal amount of polyp tissue should be captured between the jaws of the forceps (Figure 6-1). The clinician then applies tension to the handle of the forceps and the jaws are allowed to close (bite), thus capturing the tissue inside the cups of the forceps jaws themselves. Tissue is removed from the patient by simple traction (pulling) on the forceps catheter itself, and the entire device is removed from the patient so that tissue can be placed in an appropriately labeled sample jar for processing.

The polyp site should be reassessed. If residual polyp tissue is still present, additional bites should be made until complete resection is achieved. Although the risk of perforation or significant hemorrhage is low, the primary downside of this technique is that minor bleeding often occurs at the polypectomy site after the first bite. This is usually of no clinical consequence but can hinder visualization on subsequent bites.

Hot forceps polypectomy is similar to the cold forceps technique and implies the simultaneous use of electrocautery delivered to the polyp through the forceps itself during tissue removal (via traction on the forceps catheter). In general, hot forceps polypectomy should be limited to polyps smaller than 5 mm in diameter. Once the polyp is visualized and the forceps are advanced through the colonoscope, only the tip of the polyp is grasped and pulled into the lumen away from the bowel wall to create a tentlike effect. It is imperative to make the tent as narrow and elongated as possible, creating a stalklike structure out of the polyp and its associated submucosal tissue, to minimize the area subjected to the electrical current. Once this is done, the base of the polyp is cauterized and the tip remains inside the forceps to be used as a sample for pathologic examination.

A few considerations should be taken into account before cauterizing a polyp. In general, a monopolar electrocautery system with a coagulation setting is used; power should be applied at 10 to 20 W for 1 to 2 seconds.[4] Initially, it was thought that the advantage of hot forceps biopsy was the ability to minimize residual polyp tissue. However, many studies have shown that hot forceps are equivalent to cold forceps in terms of complete polyp removal.[2,5] It should be stated that, although once common, hot forceps polypectomy is rarely performed. Electrocautery can contribute significantly to complications, including bleeding, perforation, and postpolypectomy syndrome (discussed later in this chapter). Most small polyps are simply removed with cold forceps polypectomy.

Snare Polypectomy

Endoscopic snares are metal wire loops encased in a plastic sheath that can be passed through the working channel of a colonoscope. These snares can be looped around a polyp to capture the lesion, and the loop itself then can be pulled back into the sheath to close the snare. As the snare closes, the area within the loop (containing the polyp tissue) rapidly diminishes and the wires literally cut through the polyp, thus removing it from the colonic wall.

Snare polypectomy is the preferred endoscopic removal method for larger polyps. As with forceps polypectomy, snare polypectomy can be performed with or without the simultaneous use of electrocautery. The first step in snare polypectomy is selection of the appropriate snare. Endoscopic snares come in different shapes, with oval and hexagonal being the most common. Oval snares may be ideal for smaller polyps, whereas hexagonal snares are more effective when removing multiple polyps or performing piecemeal resection of a larger polyp. In addition, snares can come with a barb (an accentuated wire bend at the apex of the wire loop) that provides tissue traction when working with tissue that is difficult to capture, as in the case of flat or sessile polyps. Crescent-shaped snares are also available and can be used for endoscopic mucosal resection (EMR). Additionally, snares with a very small loop volume, known as *minisnares*, can be used to remove polyps smaller than 10 mm in diameter in lieu of a forceps polypectomy with equally good, if not better, results.[6,7] Minisnares also can be used to remove residual polyp tissue after resection of a large polyp (Figure 6-2).

Beyond the snare shape, there are also different types of snare wires. A thin monofilament wire is recommended for cold snaring and the resection of small polyps.[8] If the

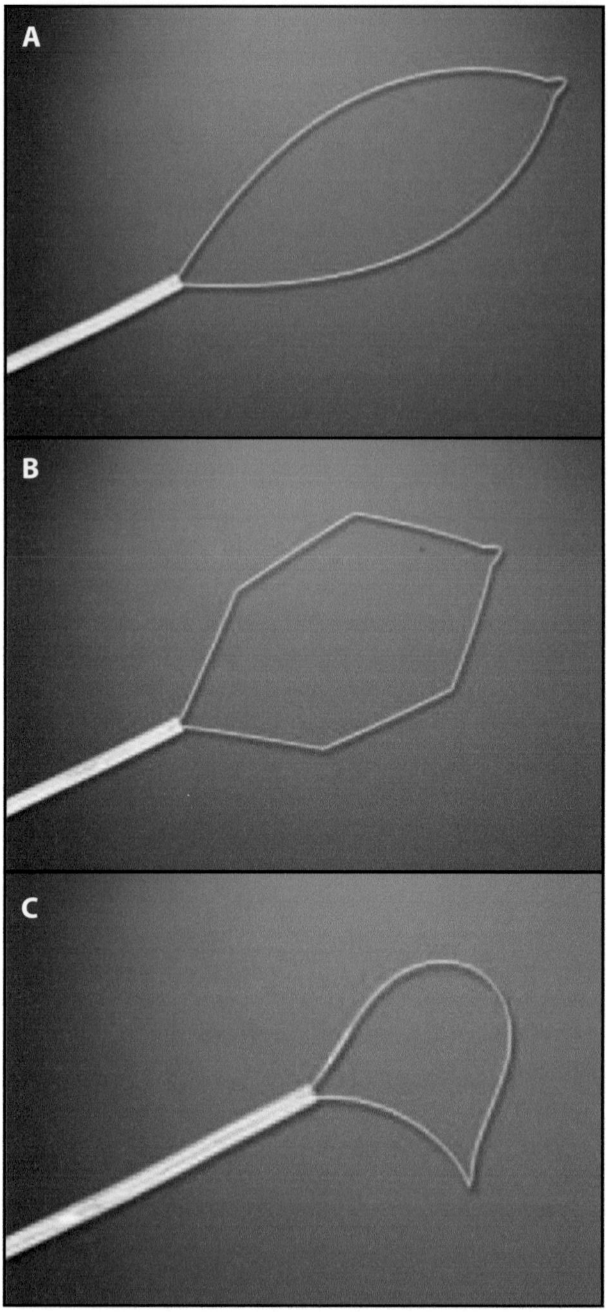

Figure 6-2. (A) An oval snare, the most commonly used snare configuration. (B) A hexagonal snare. (C) A duckbill-shaped snare. (Reprinted with permission from Cook Medical.)

decision is made to pursue a hot snare polypectomy, it is important to keep in mind that a monofilament wire promotes tissue cutting, whereas a braided wire is more likely to have a prominent coagulation effect on tissue. The most commonly used snares are braided because coagulation during snare polypectomy usually has the desired effect of reduced bleeding.

In cold snare polypectomy, electrocautery is not used and the polyp is transected by the mechanical act of closing the snare. Once the appropriate snare is selected and the polyp is brought into the 6-o'clock position, the snare is advanced through the working channel of the colonoscope. If it is difficult to loop the snare around the polyp, it can be helpful to advance the snare beyond the polyp and attempt to hook it while pulling back. After the snare is placed in position, the assistant should be instructed to close the snare until the polyp tissue is fully cut away from the luminal wall (Figures 6-3A and 6-3B). If the polyp is pedunculated, the snare should be positioned approximately halfway up the stalk. Leaving a short remnant of the polyp allows for a therapeutic target if postpolypectomy bleeding develops (Figure 6-3C).

Hot snare polypectomy is an alternative to the cold snare technique. Electrocautery is often used for polyps larger than 20 mm, broad-based polyps, polyps requiring piecemeal resection, and sessile or flat polyps. Hot snare polypectomy can also be applied effectively to smaller polyps (Figure 6-4).

Although prospective data are fairly limited regarding the most effective current to use during snare polypectomy, most gastroenterologists are equally split between modes that combine cutting and coagulation currents (referred to as *blended current*) and pure coagulation modes.[9] Both current types have been shown to have similar rates of post-polypectomy bleeding, although immediate hemorrhage was more common with blended current, and delayed hemorrhage was more common with pure coagulation current.[10] A pure cut setting is rarely used because it has been associated with higher rates of immediate postpolypectomy hemorrhage compared with blended current.[11]

Once the current is selected and the snare is advanced through the colonoscope, the polyp should be captured and then tented as far away from the colonic wall as possible. It is important to note that the snare should not be fully tightened because doing so carries a risk of inadvertently cold-cutting the polyp, which can result in excessive bleeding or entrapment of the snare within the desiccated tissue. The ideal approach is to close the snare until resistance is noted. Just as the snare is further closed and the polyp is starting to be cut, electrocautery can be applied. Morris et al[4] recommended a blended current at 20 W as the setting that optimizes both the cutting and coagulation capabilities of the electrocautery system, but the actual setting is left to the individual operator, and no gold standard exists. Some practitioners prefer lower settings on the right side of the colon where the colon wall is thinner.

Polyp Retrieval

After snare polypectomy, the resected tissue will need to be retrieved. The most common approach is to advance the colonoscope to the polyp and suction it through the accessory channel. If the polyp is too large to be suctioned en bloc, the snare can be used to cold cut it into smaller pieces; the polyp can be retrieved in a piecemeal fashion. If a polyp is to be retrieved via the suction technique, it is critical to apply a polyp trap to the endoscope to capture the specimen; failing to do so will lead to loss of the polyp. Polyp traps come in many different shapes, but all function to capture the polyp prior to its passage into the larger suction canister. Large polyps, as well as multiple large fragments, can be retrieved with the aid of a retrieval net. Retrieval nets are similar in appearance to standard snares but have an additional soft fabric mesh netting that can grasp material much like an insect net.

If the polyp disappears from view after snare resection, the water bolus method can aid in retrieval.[12] In this method, the colonoscope is placed at the polypectomy site and the

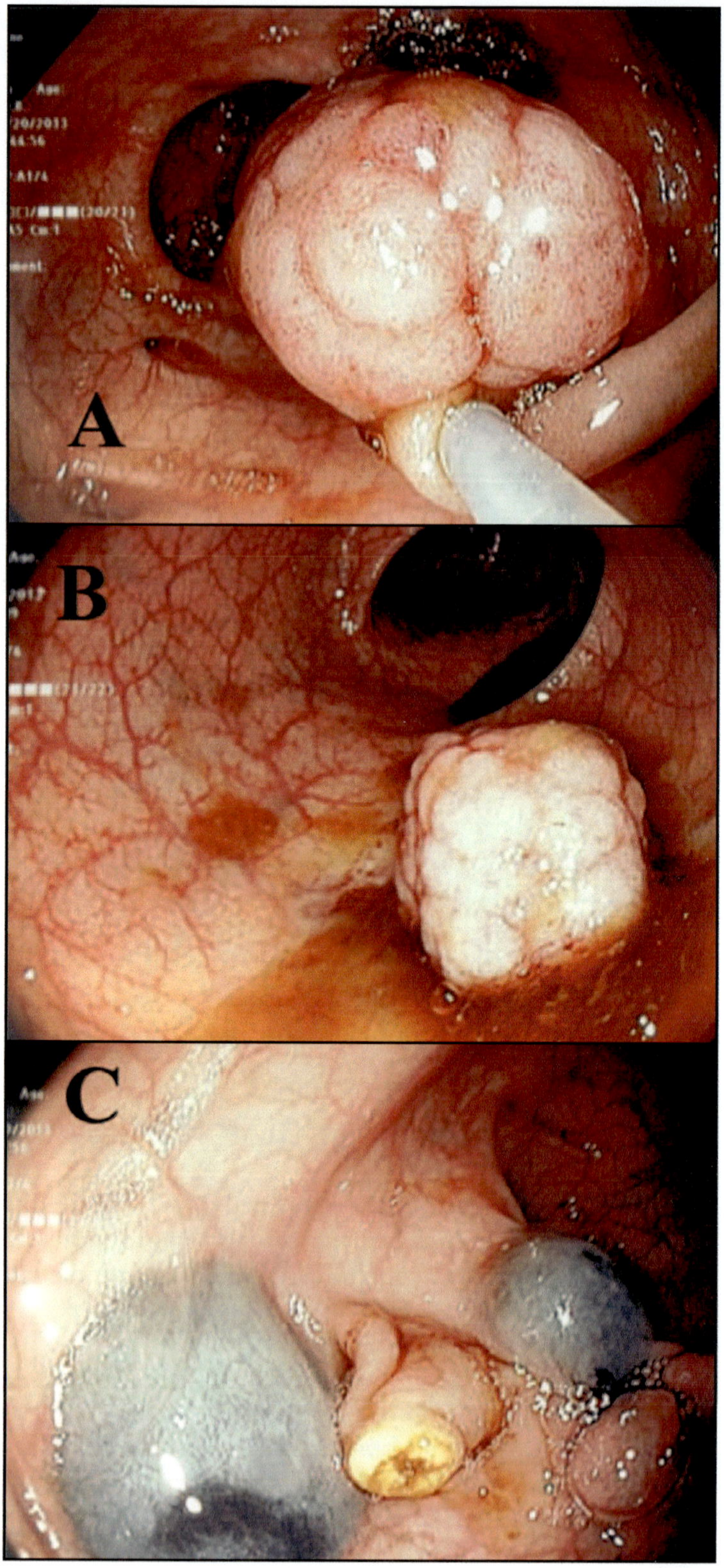

Figure 6-3. (A) A 4-cm pedunculated polyp identified in the sigmoid. An endoscopic snare was placed around the polyp's stalk halfway between the colon wall and the polyp itself. (B) The polyp was then removed by closing the snare. The excised polyp was then free within the colonic lumen. Before resection, this polyp was injected with epinephrine in an attempt to shrink the lesion. (C) A small residual stalk. It is not bleeding, but if it were, there was adequate stalk tissue to grasp and treat with cautery or clips. The polyp site was tattooed for future reference. The pathologic examination revealed tubulovillous adenoma. (Reprinted with permission from Serag Dredar, MD.)

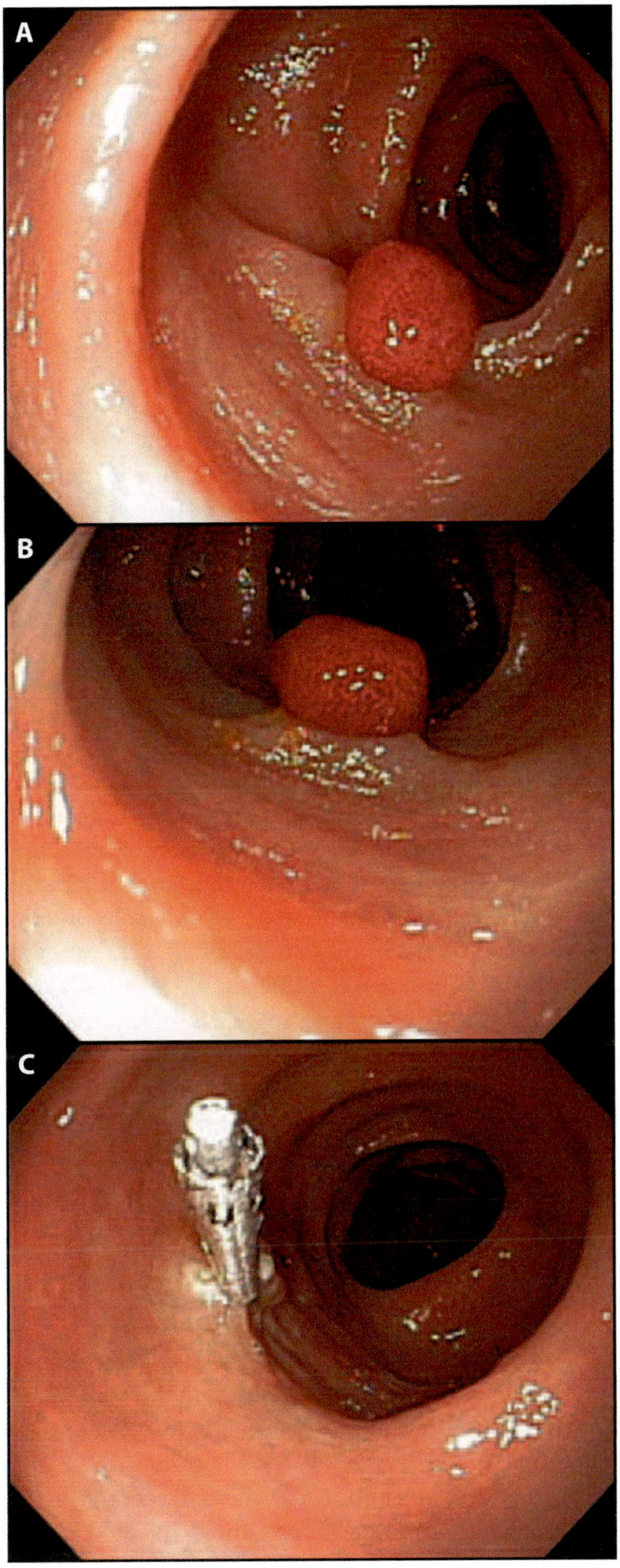

Figure 6-4. (A) A sessile polyp found during colonoscopy. (B) The polyp had a somewhat wide base, and a hot snare was used to remove the lesion despite its somewhat small size. (C) The site of the polypectomy after endoscopic application of a clip to minimize the risk of postpolypectomy bleeding. (Reprinted with permission of Douglas G. Adler, MD, FACG, AGAF, FASGE.)

clinician injects a small bolus of water. If the stream of water moves away from the visual field, that means gravity has taken the tissue proximal to the polypectomy site and the scope should be advanced to the first pool of water, where the polyp will likely be found. Alternatively, if water appears to be streaming over the visual field, the opposite would hold true and the polyp should be searched for distal to the polypectomy site.

Advanced Techniques

Submucosal Cushion

Submucosal cushion, also known as *injection-assisted polypectomy*, is a technique that involves injecting a liquid substance into the submucosal space to raise the polyp into the lumen and facilitate its resection. This technique may decrease the risk of perforation, bleeding, and thermal injury to surrounding colonic tissue by creating a submucosal cushion that acts as a buffer between the polypectomy itself and the deeper layers of the colonic wall. This method is frequently used to resect sessile or flat polyps larger than 15 mm in diameter, as well as polyps located on top of mucosal folds.

The most common fluid used for injection is normal saline, either on its own or in combination with epinephrine or methylene blue. The advantages of saline are its low cost, widespread availability, and safety. When saline is combined with adrenaline, the solution also serves to shrink the polyp and induce vasoconstriction, thus minimizing bleeding during the resection. The disadvantage of the injection of saline alone is that it dissipates quickly, especially in highly vascularized areas of the bowel, such as the rectum, which means the cushion may not persist long enough for one to accomplish the entire resection and additional injections may be required. It should be noted that the vasoconstrictive effects of the norepinephrine can lead to ischemia of the bowel wall, although in practice this is rare. Therefore, in the parts of the colon with thinner walls, such as the cecum, epinephrine should be diluted to at least 1:100 000 or normal saline should be used alone.

Alternative fluids for submucosal injection include normal saline with methylene blue, indigo carmine, dextrose, autologous blood or packed red blood cells from the patient, hypertonic saline, and hyaluronic acid; the latter 2 are associated with local tissue inflammation. Although hyaluronic acid has been shown to create the longest-lasting cushion, it also was found to be associated with tumor cell proliferation in artificial wounds in a murine model.[13] Recent studies have also shown that dextrose 50% was superior to normal saline in maintaining the submucosal cushion and facilitating resection, particularly of large, sessile polyps.[14,15] Researchers in these studies also observed an increased risk of postpolypectomy syndrome among patients treated with dextrose. In clinical practice, simple saline is the most commonly used fluid for creating a submucosal cushion. A small amount of indigo carmine may be added to normal saline to lift the polyp. The blue tinge obtained helps better identify the polyp borders and highlights the underlying submucosa after resection. In the uncommon scenario of perforation, an endoscopic target sign can be better appreciated when this dye is used.

When creating the cushion, the goal is to inject the fluid below the polyp between the submucosal and mucosal layers to help separate them. The polyp can be injected on the distal or proximal side. If the distal side is injected before the proximal side, the polyp may tilt away from the colonoscope and can make any additional injections more difficult. If the clinician has significant difficulty when trying to inject the proximal portion of the polyp, retroflexion (if deemed safe to perform in that location) can be attempted to facilitate the process. The needle then should be advanced out of the scope and directed toward the base of the polyp almost tangentially to the mucosa (ie, the angle should be less than 30 degrees). Once the needle is positioned properly, it should be advanced an additional 2 to 3 mm below the surface of the mucosa into the top part of the submucosa.[8,16] Injection of the solution should be initiated slowly as the needle is retracted back from the bowel wall. Usually 2 to 4 mL is sufficient for one to attain an appropriately sized cushion, although more or less fluid may be needed, depending on the size and shape of the polyp. Some experts recommend beginning injection immediately prior to advancing the needle into the polyp base, which allows for the solution to find the submucosal space. With this technique, needle advancement is stopped once lifting of the polyp is noted.

If additional injections are necessary, the best approach is to perform subsequent injections at the lateral edge of a previously formed cushion. Failure of the polyp to lift may represent insertion of the needle through the mucosa and into the peritoneum. Alternatively, this may represent submucosal fibrosis related to an underlying malignant lesion.[17] The most frequent cause of a failure to lift is a previous attempt at endoscopic resection that has led to submucosal fibrosis. A nonlifting sign may be a signal to abort attempts at polypectomy altogether and refer the patient to a surgeon. Once the polyp has been lifted adequately, it can be snared off in a hot or cold manner, and any resulting tissue defect can be clipped if needed (Figure 6-5).

Endoscopic Mucosal Resection

EMR refers to an aggressive polypectomy, which attempts to remove a lesion in its entirety with the goal of clearing all margins. This technique has been developed as a surgical alternative for the management of polyps not amenable to conventional snare or forceps polypectomy, including broad-based pedunculated, sessile, and flat lesions (Figure 6-6). EMR can be performed either as a single resection or in a piecemeal manner, with the latter indicated for sessile or flat polyps that are usually larger than 20 mm in diameter.

The initial step of EMR is the creation of a submucosal cushion. This submucosal cushion ensures that the polyp is raised adequately away from the submucosa, thus minimizing the risk of perforation and thermal injury from the use of electrocautery, which may be repetitive if one is performing a piecemeal resection. In fact, it may be more effective to create a cushion under one portion of the polyp, resect it, and then repeat the same process with the next portion of the lesion; this way, the submucosal cushion will not have time to dissipate before the resection is done. EMR is one scenario where using the pure cut or Endocut (ERBE Corporation) setting may be advantageous because the lower voltage of these currents decreases the extent of tissue trauma. Once the appropriate cushion is created, a hot snare is used to perform the resection. Initially, a large snare can be used to grasp larger pieces of the lesion, with remaining portions being resected with smaller, barbed, or spiral snares. An example of EMR for removal of a large sessile polyp is demonstrated in Video 6-1.

If EMR is complicated by the fact that the polyp has a large head, a process called *epinephrine volume reduction* can be done (see Figure 6-1). A study by Hogan et al[18] demonstrated the effectiveness of this technique in large, pedunculated polyps. They injected 4 to 8 mL epinephrine (1:10 000) into several sites in the head of the polyp and then another 2 to 4 mL into the polyp stalk. After a wait time of 3 to 5 minutes, researchers

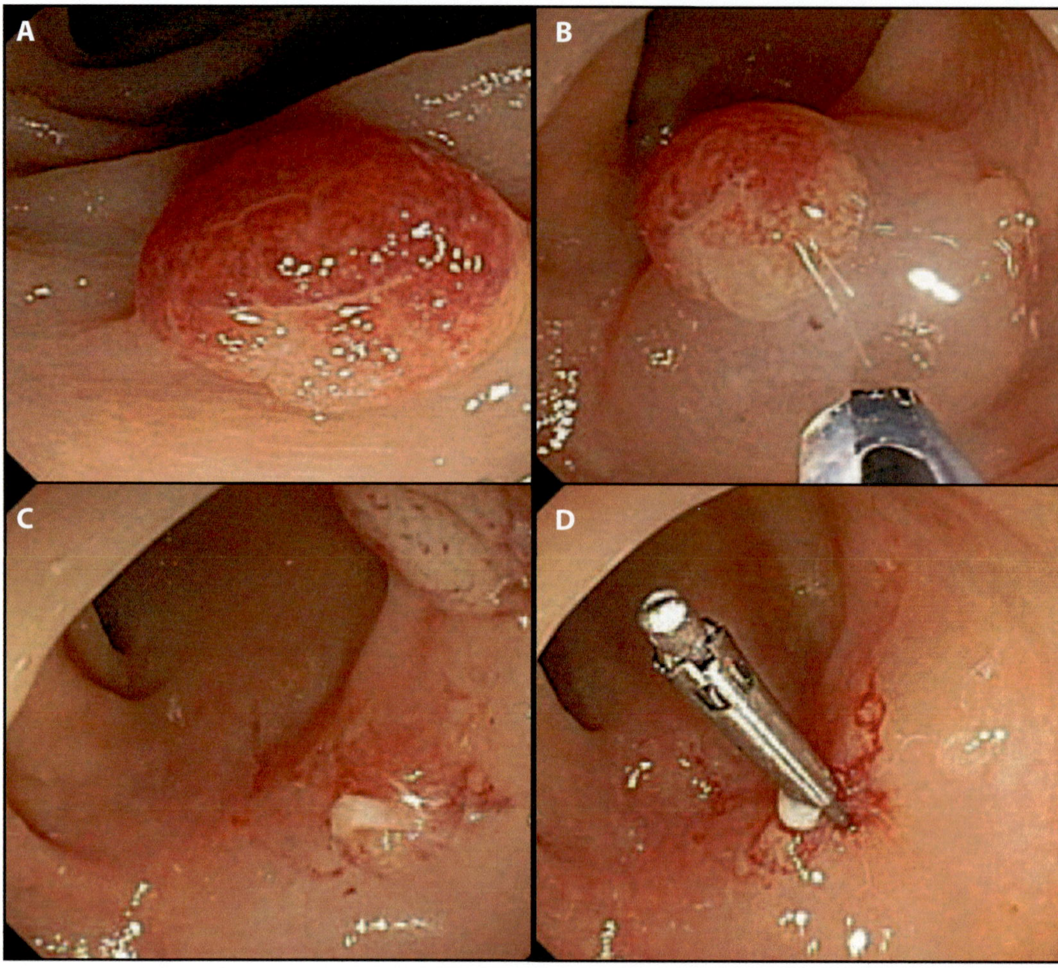

Figure 6-5. (A) A medium-sized sessile polyp. (B) With a combined snare/needle device, a submucosal cushion was created using the needle to lift the polyp into the lumen. (C) The appearance of the site after removal of the lesion with hot snare polypectomy. (D) A single clip was applied to the site prophylactically. (Reprinted with permission of Douglas G. Adler, MD, FACG, AGAF, FASGE.)

observed a significant reduction in the polyp size resulting from vasoconstriction, and this often facilitated resection of the polyp in one piece with minimal postprocedural bleeding. It is important to note that this technique was used only on pedunculated polyps with relatively spherical heads.

Despite its advantages, EMR is not always successful in completely removing a large polyp. If residual tissue remains, argon plasma coagulation (APC) has been shown to be an effective adjunct to incomplete polypectomy. The major advantage of APC is that it can be performed either immediately after the resection as a means of removing endoscopically visible tissue or on a repeat colonoscopy to remove any tissue that remained or has regrown since the last procedure.[16,19] If the polyp is sessile, has advanced histologic findings, or prompts concerns about incomplete removal, a follow-up colonoscopy should be performed within the next several months to ensure complete polyp resection.

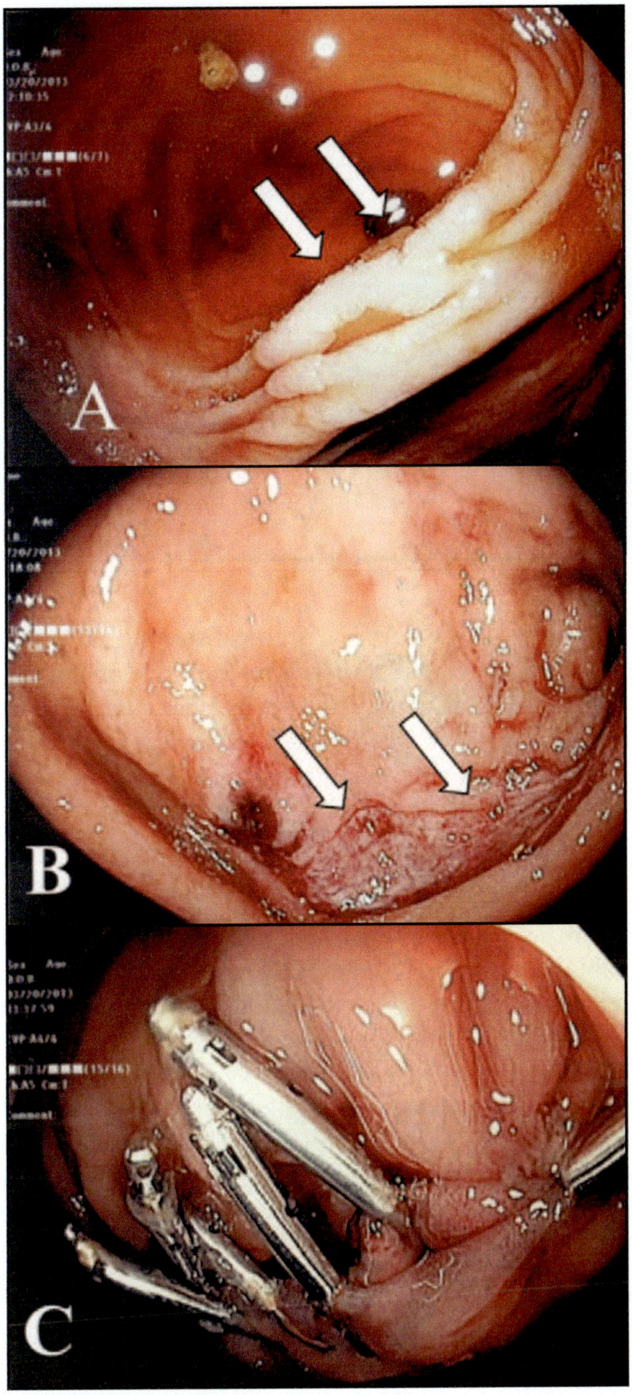

Figure 6-6. (A) A flat sessile polyp measuring 2 cm in length is identified in the cecum. It can be seen to involve 3 of the periappendiceal folds. It was lifted using normal saline and was resected using a snare. (B) The polyp was removed with EMR, leaving a broad, irregular mucosal defect. (C) The defect was then closed using endoscopic clips. The pathologic examination confirmed tubular adenoma. (Reprinted with permission from Serag Dredar, MD.)

Endoscopic Submucosal Dissection

Endoscopic submucosal dissection (ESD) is a fairly new and aggressive method for resecting colonic polyps in a single piece. This technique is indicated for removing large sessile or lateral spreading lesions, where the suspicion of malignancy is high. The main technical difference between ESD and en bloc EMR is the use of various endoscopic

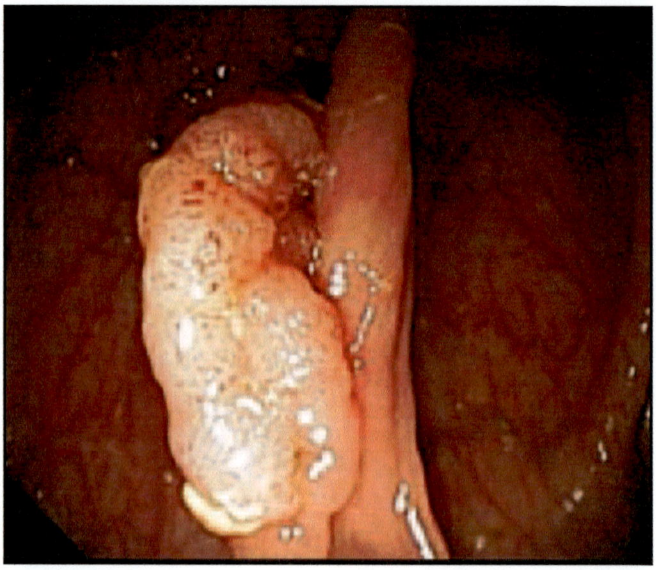

Figure 6-7. A sessile polyp along a fold that may be difficult to remove without a submucosal cushion. (Reprinted with permission of Douglas G. Adler, MD, FACG, AGAF, FASGE.)

knives to execute the resection. Additionally, ESD is more time consuming and may require several hours to complete. ESD is also associated with a significant rate of complications, most notably perforation. Currently, ESD is used primarily in Japan and Europe, with only a handful of US endoscopy centers offering this technique. However, as expertise in ESD continues to increase and complication rates decline, the procedure will likely become more prevalent in the United States as well.

Colonic Tattooing

Tattooing with India ink can be used in several situations. When endoscopic resection of the polyp is incomplete or not feasible, a tattoo may help one identify the polyp site for future endoscopic or surgical resection procedures. Such situations include very large polyps in the cecum, where the risk of perforation is high; ulcerated lesions concerning for invasive malignancy; and piecemeal EMR that may leave residual polyp tissue behind. In the first 2 situations, tattooing allows for fairly accurate polyp localization during surgical intervention, thus minimizing the need for intraoperative colonoscopy.[20,21] In the instance of piecemeal EMR, surveillance often is necessary after the initial resection to monitor for residual tissue, and tattooing can be helpful in reidentifying the site of the original polyp.

Miscellaneous Techniques

A polypectomy can be complicated not just by the size or shape of the lesion, but also by its location within the colon. If a polyp is located on top of a mucosal fold (Figure 6-7), it is important to create a submucosal cushion before the resection to reduce the risk of perforation. If the polyp is hiding behind a fold and is difficult to reach, a double-channel colonoscope can be used with a grasper advanced through one of the channels and the snare advanced through the other. The grasper then can be used to grab the polyp and manipulate it into the snare. Alternatively, 10 to 40 mL saline can be injected into the lumen proximal to the polyp with the idea that the water bolus will push the polyp out of its hiding place and into better view.[22] Another option is to attach a plastic cap to the tip of the colonoscope and use it to push down and straighten the fold obstructing access to the polyp.[22]

Access to polyps on the proximal side of folds also can be improved by performing colonic retroflexion at locations other than in the rectum. This technique has been demonstrated to be effective and safe in all segments of the colon when one is using a pediatric colonoscope and can sometimes be performed with an adult instrument.[23] In a situation where the polyp is difficult to bring into view because it is located on an inaccessible part of the colon wall, a side-viewing instrument such as a duodenoscope can be helpful for one to clearly visualize and remove the lesion. If colonic peristalsis moves the polyp in and out of the visual field, intravenous glucagon or hyoscyamine can be given to relieve the excessive motility. Finally, basic techniques such as repositioning the patient or compressing the abdomen can help manipulate the bowel wall and, as a result, bring the polyp into a better position.

Avoiding Complications

As many as one-third of all patients report benign and short-lived symptoms such as abdominal pain, bloating, small amounts of lower gastrointestinal bleeding, nausea, and diarrhea after a colonoscopy.[24] Serious complications such as profound bleeding, colonic perforation, and postpolypectomy electrocoagulation syndrome (PPECS) represent potential risks of which the patient and endoscopist should be aware. A review of 57,000 colonoscopies found that serious adverse events occurred in approximately 2.8 per 1000 colonoscopies.[25] More than 85% of these serious complications were reported in patients who had colonoscopy with polypectomy. Although there are risks in colonoscopy with polypectomy, the overall mortality rate has been reported as extremely low, between 0.007% and 0.03%.[24,26] Specific quality indicators (QIs) have been proposed by several gastroenterology societies, including the American Society for Gastrointestinal Endoscopy (ASGE) and the United Kingdom National Health Service Bowel Cancer Screening Programme (UK NHS-BCSP), to promote tracking of success, failure, and complication rates.[27,28] Some of the more serious complications are reviewed next.

Bleeding

According to the ASGE, polypectomy is considered a high-risk procedure.[29] The incidence of postpolypectomy hemorrhage is between 0.3% and 6%, but rates as high as 24% have been reported in patients undergoing endoscopic removal of larger polyps.[30]

There are 2 types of postpolypectomy bleeding: immediate (recognized by the endoscopist during the procedure) and delayed (identified as long as 1 month after polypectomy). The incidence of immediate bleeding after polypectomy has been reported to be 1.5% to 2.8%.[11,31,32] Risk factors for immediate bleeding include patient age greater than 65 years, comorbid cardiovascular or kidney disease, polyps larger than 1 cm, the use of cut or blended electrocautery, the presence of pedunculated or laterally spreading polyps, poor bowel preparation, and certain anticoagulation medications.[11] Delayed bleeding has been reported in as many as 2% of polypectomies, and risk factors include the use of coagulation current and the presence of hypertension.[33,34] The QI standard for postpolypectomy bleeding has been set at less than 1% by the ASGE and UK NHS-BCSP.[27,28]

Optimizing a patient's coagulation status before polypectomy is an important step in avoiding postpolypectomy bleeding. Multiple retrospective studies found no association between the use of aspirin or other nonsteroidal anti-inflammatory drugs and an increased risk of postpolypectomy bleeding.[35,36] In contrast, warfarin appears to increase postpolypectomy bleeding as much as 13-fold at both therapeutic and subtherapeutic doses.[35] Depending on the indication for anticoagulation, warfarin can either be withheld for 3 to 5 days before the procedure or bridged with heparin.[37] There are also limited data on the prophylactic use of endoclips in patients taking antithrombotic medications.[38] The amount of time that anticoagulation needs to be withheld after polypectomy can be individualized.

During the past several years, numerous new oral anticoagulant medications have been approved by the US Food and Drug Administration, including the direct thrombin inhibitor dabigatran (Pradaxa) and factor Xa inhibitors rivaroxaban (Xarelto) and apixaban (Eliquis). Dabigatran should be withheld for at least 1 to 2 days before polypectomy in patients with a glomerular filtration rate (GFR) greater than 50 mL/min and at least 3 to 5 days in patients with a GFR less than 50 mL/min. The risks and benefits of withholding rivaroxaban and apixaban before polypectomy should be weighed carefully given their black box warning of increased risk of stroke in patients with nonvalvular atrial fibrillation on discontinuation. Therefore, one should consider cardiology and/or hematology consultation before these new anticoagulants are withheld.

Injection of epinephrine (1:10000) into both pedunculated and sessile polyps before removal is commonly performed to reduce bleeding, although there are conflicting data regarding its effect on postpolypectomy bleeding. A small randomized trial showed that the injection of epinephrine into polyps produced an 8 times lower risk of immediate bleeding compared with standard polypectomies.[39] A larger study conducted by Lee et al[40] reported no significant difference in any type of postpolypectomy bleeding when comparing epinephrine injection with the standard polypectomy technique.

Endoloops are detachable snares that can be placed around the polyp base or stalk and then tightened before the polypectomy is performed.[41] They have been shown to decrease postpolypectomy bleeding compared with the standard technique in polyps at least 1 to 2 cm or larger.[42,43] Epinephrine injection and endoloops also have been used in combination, showing a statistically significant decrease in bleeding risk compared with epinephrine injection alone.[44] Endoclips can also be applied to the base of a polyp or across a stalk before resection in an attempt to prevent postpolypectomy bleeding, although extra caution must be exercised to ensure current is not applied to the metal endoclip to prevent the risk of burning or perforating the colonic wall (Figure 6-8).[45]

Colonic Perforation

The colonic perforation rate during resection of polyps smaller than 2 cm is between 0.3% and 0.5% and as high as 1.3% for those larger than 2 cm.[31,46] If ESD is used, the perforation rates have been reported to be as high as 10%.[16] Although the overall incidence is low, colonic perforation carries a relatively high risk of mortality, which is as high as 5%.[47] The ASGE and UK NHS-BCSP have set the QI standard for colonic perforation at less than 1/500 for all colonoscopies and less than 1/1000 for screening colonoscopies.[27,28] Colonic perforations are often caused by excessive pressure within the colon, mechanical trauma applied by the colonoscope to the colonic wall, or electrocautery. Risk factors during polypectomy include larger polyps, sessile polyps, polyps located in the proximal colon

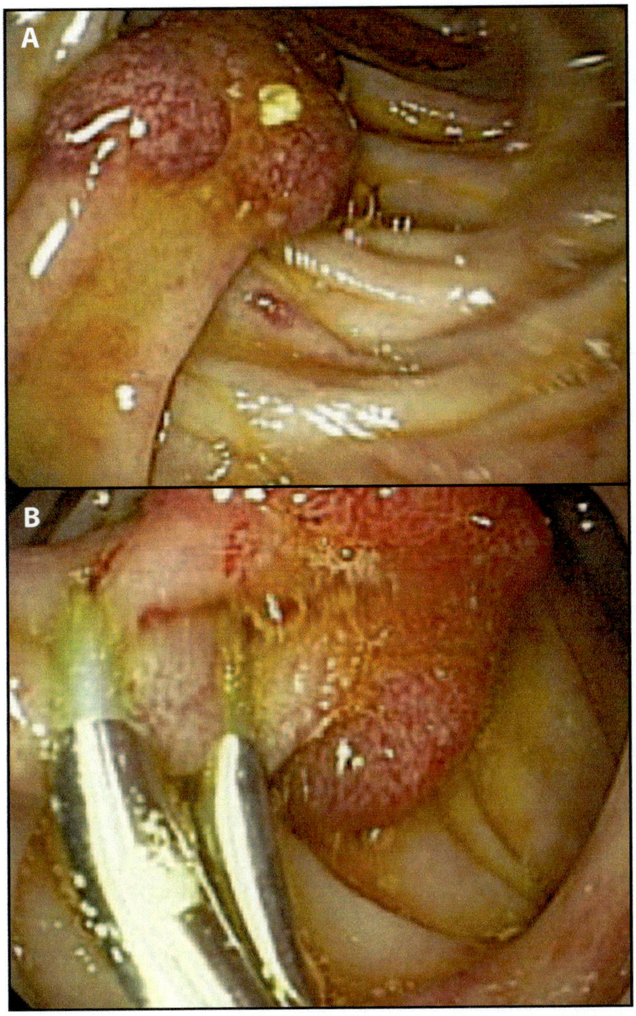

Figure 6-8. (A) A pedunculated polyp with a thick stalk that was believed likely to harbor a significant vessel. (B) The same polyp after prophylactic placement of 2 endoscopic clips across the lesion before attempts at removal to minimize the risk of bleeding. (Reprinted with permission of Douglas G. Adler, MD, FACG, AGAF, FASGE.)

(secondary to a thinner wall), history of diverticular disease, longer electrocautery times, and the endoscopist's level of experience.[26,47]

Some basic approaches can be used to avoid colonic perforation. Replacing oxygen with carbon dioxide for insufflation and using a colonoscope with lower maximum air flow rates (if available) can reduce the pressure within the colon.[48] Electrocautery using the cut current also has been associated with a higher risk of perforation as compared with blended and coagulation settings.[41,49] Cold forceps and cold snaring techniques can be used to remove smaller polyps to avoid electrocautery and minimize the risk of perforation. The use of cold snaring during polypectomy has an almost insignificant risk of perforation while providing quality specimens compared with hot biopsy.[49,50]

Postpolypectomy Electrocoagulation Syndrome

PPECS is a constellation of symptoms resulting from the electrical current applied to the colonic wall during a polypectomy. The current causes a transmural burn that extends through the mucosa, muscularis propria, and serosa. There is no frank perforation; instead, an inflammatory reaction is causing a more localized peritonitis. Risk factors for

PPECS are removal of polyps larger than 2 cm and increased duration of applied electric current.[41] Techniques similar to those used to avoid perforation can also be used to limit PPECS, including using caution with the type and duration of electrocautery current.

Managing Complications

Bleeding

General management of bleeding includes an order that the patient receive nothing by mouth, initiating intravenous fluids, checking serial hemoglobin levels, and maintaining an active blood type and screen because approximately 50% of patients arriving at the hospital with hematochezia after polypectomy will require a blood transfusion.[36] Additionally, surgery or interventional radiology consultations should be considered if there is concern that hemostasis may not be established by endoscopic means.

Endoscopic Management

Immediate bleeding identified during the polypectomy can be stopped by applying pressure with the snare or forceps tip. Epinephrine injection to the bleeding site can also facilitate the cessation of bleeding. Electrocautery to the bleeding site is another common approach, and current should be administered in multiple, short intervals rather than a prolonged, continuous flow to achieve better hemostasis and safety. Endoclips alone or in combination with APC can be used for both pedunculated and sessile polyps.[51,52] Endoloops can be especially useful in providing hemostasis in resected pedunculated polyps that have long pedicles. Band ligation has been used for significant immediate or delayed bleeding after polypectomy, although high suction pressures should be avoided, especially in the right colon.[53,54]

Angiography and Surgical Management

Angiographic control of postpolypectomy bleeding can be considered an alternative to surgery in a patient with recurrent or severe bleeding refractory to endoscopic interventions. A tagged red blood cell scan can assist in identifying the location of the bleed if the hemorrhage is active and brisk enough.[55] The optimal clinical conditions for angiography include an international normalized ratio less than 1.5, platelet count greater than 50,000, serum creatinine level less than 1.5 mg/dL, and GFR greater than 60 mL/min.[56] If the patient's coagulation status is not optimal, fresh-frozen plasma and/or platelets should be available before or during the procedure. Angiographic therapies include embolization of the actively bleeding vessel or administration of vasopressin. If endoscopic and angiographic interventions are unsuccessful, then surgical intervention should be considered.

Colonic Perforation

Patients in whom colonic perforation develops after polypectomy are usually seen with moderate to severe abdominal pain, fever, tachycardia, and leukocytosis. On physical examination, the patient can have findings consistent with peritonitis, such as rebound tenderness, guarding, and distension. There should be a low threshold to image a patient with a suspected colonic perforation, with an upright chest and abdominal radiograph to rule out free air. If no free air is seen and there is still a high suspicion for perforation, a computed tomography scan of the abdomen can demonstrate intraperitoneal and retroperitoneal air with greater sensitivity.[49] The lack of free air on imaging does not preclude the need for surgery if the clinical suspicion for perforation is still high.

Conservative Management

Conservative management in patients found to have colonic perforation initially begins with bowel rest (nothing by mouth), intravenous fluids, and antibiotics. Antibiotic coverage should target gram-negative and anaerobic organisms. Surgical consultation should be considered if a perforation is suspected. Conservative medical therapy has a reported success rate ranging between 33% and 85%, especially for microperforations.[49,57] Patients who have an adequate bowel preparation and minimal peritoneal signs or symptoms on examination can show improvement during the initial 24 hours and have the best outcomes with conservative therapy.[58]

Endoscopic Management

Depending on the perforation size and the experience and skill of the endoscopist, some perforations can be closed endoscopically if they are visualized immediately. The ideal perforation for endoscopic closure is less than 10 mm.[59,60] The application of one or more endoclips allows for a relatively conservative medical approach while at the same time promoting tissue healing. A review of 75 perforations repaired by endoclip placement reported a success rate between 69% and 93%.[60]

Surgical Management

If a patient's condition does not improve after 24 to 48 hours of conservative or endoscopic treatment or the patient has overt signs of perforation such as significant peritonitis, then surgery should be considered as first-line management. If the perforation involves greater than 50% of the bowel circumference, simple primary closure can be performed.[61] For larger perforations, bowel resection with either primary anastomosis or diversion may be needed. Perforation repair via laparoscopy has been shown to reduce length of stay, has fewer postoperative complications, and requires a smaller surgical incision.[62] Postoperative morbidity and mortality have been reported to be as high as 24% and 5.4%, respectively, if diagnosis is delayed, with comorbidities contributing to a higher mortality rate.[49]

Postpolypectomy Electrocoagulation Syndrome

Management for PPECS is typically conservative and consists of ordering nothing by mouth for the patient and administering intravenous fluids and either oral or intravenous antibiotics. Approximately 20% of patients will need to be admitted to the hospital to receive this treatment, whereas most patients with mild symptoms can be treated as outpatients.[32] Patients typically improve within 24 hours and should have near-complete cessation of symptoms with treatment within 4 days.[49] If there is a high suspicion for perforation, imaging can be performed to differentiate between the 2 conditions. Unlike patients with true colonic perforation, patients with PPECS will not have evidence of free air, although the lack of free air does not definitively rule out perforation or the need for surgery.

Conclusion

Endoscopic polypectomy of colon polyps is an important technique that every endoscopist should master. The process should always begin with the assessment of the polyp features to determine the best resection method to minimize the risk of complications. There are no explicit guidelines indicating how to approach any given polyp, and it is frequently up to the endoscopist's discretion and expertise. It is important to remember that large polyps pose a higher risk of bleeding and perforation and should be resected with particular care. Also, not all polyps are endoscopically resectable even by the most experienced gastroenterologist. If such a lesion is encountered, it is not unreasonable to refer the patient for a surgical consult.

References

1. Edwards BK, Ward E, Kohler BA, et al. Annual report to the nation on the status of cancer, 1975-2006, featuring colorectal cancer trends and impact of interventions (risk factors, screening, and treatment) to reduce future rates. *Cancer.* 2010;116:544-573.
2. Draganov PV, Chang MN, Alkhasawneh A, et al. Randomized, controlled trial of standard, large-capacity versus jumbo biopsy forceps for polypectomy of small, sessile, colorectal polyps. *Gastrointest Endosc.* 2012;75:118-126.
3. Efthymiou M, Taylor AC, Desmond PV, Allen PB, Chen RY. Biopsy forceps is inadequate for the resection of diminutive polyps. *Endoscopy.* 2011;43:312-316.
4. Morris ML, Tucker RD, Baron TH, Song LM. Electrosurgery in gastrointestinal endoscopy: principles to practice. *Am J Gastroenterol.* 2009;104:1563-1574.
5. Vanagunas A, Jacob P, Vakil N. Adequacy of "hot biopsy" for the treatment of diminutive polyps: a prospective randomized trial. *Am J Gastroenterol.* 1989;84:383-385.
6. McAfee JH, Katon RM. Tiny snares prove safe and effective for removal of diminutive colorectal polyps. *Gastrointest Endosc.* 1994;40:301-303.
7. Uno Y, Obara K, Zheng P, et al. Cold snare excision is a safe method for diminutive colorectal polyps. *Tohoku J Exp Med.* 1997;183:243-249.
8. Monkemuller K, Neumann H, Malfertheiner P, Fry LC. Advanced colon polypectomy. *Clin Gastroenterol Hepatol.* 2009;7:641-652.
9. Singh N, Harrison M, Rex DK. A survey of colonoscopic polypectomy practices among clinical gastroenterologists. *Gastrointest Endosc.* 2004;60:414-418.
10. Van GA, Cozzoli A, Adler M, Taton G, Cremer M. Colonoscopic snare polypectomy: analysis of 1485 resections comparing two types of current. *Gastrointest Endosc.* 1992;38:472-475.
11. Kim HS, Kim TI, Kim WH, et al. Risk factors for immediate postpolypectomy bleeding of the colon: a multicenter study. *Am J Gastroenterol.* 2006;101:1333-1341.
12. Waye J. It ain't over 'til it's over: retrieval of polyps after colonoscopic polypectomy. *Gastrointest Endosc.* 2005;62:257-259.
13. Matsui Y, Inomata M, Izumi K, Sonoda K, Shiraishi N, Kitano S. Hyaluronic acid stimulates tumor-cell proliferation at wound sites. *Gastrointest Endosc.* 2004;60:539-543.
14. Katsinelos P, Kountouras J, Paroutoglou G, et al. A comparative study of 50% dextrose and normal saline solution on their ability to create submucosal fluid cushions for endoscopic resection of sessile rectosigmoid polyps. *Gastrointest Endosc.* 2008;68:692-698.
15. Varadarajulu S, Tamhane A, Slaughter RL. Evaluation of dextrose 50% as a medium for injection-assisted polypectomy. *Endoscopy.* 2006;38:907-912.
16. Vormbrock K, Monkemuller K. Difficult colon polypectomy. *World J Gastrointest Endosc.* 2012;4:269-280.
17. Uno Y, Munakata A. The non-lifting sign of invasive colon cancer. *Gastrointest Endosc.* 1994;40:485-489.
18. Hogan RB, Hogan RB III. Epinephrine volume reduction of giant colon polyps facilitates endoscopic assessment and removal. *Gastrointest Endosc.* 2007;66:1018-1022.

19. Regula J, Wronska E, Polkowski M, et al. Argon plasma coagulation after piecemeal polypectomy of sessile colorectal adenomas: long-term follow-up study. *Endoscopy.* 2003;35:212-218.
20. Cho YB, Lee WY, Yun HR, Lee WS, Yun SH, Chun HK. Tumor localization for laparoscopic colorectal surgery. *World J Surg.* 2007;31:1491-1495.
21. Feingold DL, Addona T, Forde KA, et al. Safety and reliability of tattooing colorectal neoplasms prior to laparoscopic resection. *J Gastrointest Surg.* 2004;8:543-546.
22. Friedland S. Optimizing resection of difficult colon polyps. *Gastrointest Endosc.* 2006;63:148-149.
23. Rex DK, Khashab M. Colonoscopic polypectomy in retroflexion. *Gastrointest Endosc.* 2006;63:144-148.
24. Ko CW, Dominitz JA. Complications of colonoscopy: magnitude and management. *Gastrointest Endosc Clin N Am.* 2010;20:659-671.
25. Whitlock EP, Lin JS, Liles E, Beil TL, Fu R. Screening for colorectal cancer: a targeted, updated systematic review for the U.S. Preventive Services Task Force. *Ann Intern Med.* 2008;149:638-658.
26. Rabeneck L, Paszat LF, Hilsden RJ, et al. Bleeding and perforation after outpatient colonoscopy and their risk factors in usual clinical practice. *Gastroenterology.* 2008;135:1899-1906.
27. Choo WK, Subhani J. Complication rates of colonic polypectomy in relation to polyp characteristics and techniques: a district hospital experience. *J Interv Gastroenterol.* 2012;2:8-11.
28. Rex DK, Petrini JL, Baron TH, et al. Quality indicators for colonoscopy. *Gastrointest Endosc.* 2006;63:S16-S28.
29. Anderson MA, Ben-Menachem T, Gan SI, et al. Management of antithrombotic agents for endoscopic procedures. *Gastrointest Endosc.* 2009;70:1060-1070.
30. Dobrowolski S, Dobosz M, Babicki A, Glowacki J, Nalecz A. Blood supply of colorectal polyps correlates with risk of bleeding after colonoscopic polypectomy. *Gastrointest Endosc.* 2006;63:1004-1009.
31. Consolo P, Luigiano C, Strangio G, et al. Efficacy, risk factors and complications of endoscopic polypectomy: ten year experience at a single center. *World J Gastroenterol.* 2008;14:2364-2369.
32. Waye JD, Lewis BS, Yessayan S. Colonoscopy: a prospective report of complications. *J Clin Gastroenterol.* 1992;15:347-351.
33. Sorbi D, Norton I, Conio M, Balm R, Zinsmeister A, Gostout CJ. Postpolypectomy lower GI bleeding: descriptive analysis. *Gastrointest Endosc.* 2000;51:690-696.
34. Watabe H, Yamaji Y, Okamoto M, et al. Risk assessment for delayed hemorrhagic complication of colonic polypectomy: polyp-related factors and patient-related factors. *Gastrointest Endosc.* 2006;64:73-78.
35. Hui AJ, Wong RM, Ching JY, Hung LC, Chung SC, Sung JJ. Risk of colonoscopic polypectomy bleeding with anticoagulants and antiplatelet agents: analysis of 1657 cases. *Gastrointest Endosc.* 2004;59:44-48.
36. Sawhney MS, Salfiti N, Nelson DB, Lederle FA, Bond JH. Risk factors for severe delayed postpolypectomy bleeding. *Endoscopy.* 2008;40:115-119.
37. Fuster V, Ryden LE, Cannom DS, et al. ACC/AHA/ESC 2006 guidelines for the management of patients with atrial fibrillation: full text: a report of the American College of Cardiology/American Heart Association Task Force on practice guidelines and the European Society of Cardiology Committee for Practice Guidelines (Writing Committee to Revise the 2001 Guidelines for the Management of Patients with Atrial Fibrillation) developed in collaboration with the European Heart Rhythm Association and the Heart Rhythm Society. *Europace.* 2006;8:651-745.
38. Friedland S, Sedehi D, Soetikno R. Colonoscopic polypectomy in anticoagulated patients. *World J Gastroenterol.* 2009;15:1973-1976.
39. Dobrowolski S, Dobosz M, Babicki A, Dymecki D, Hac S. Prophylactic submucosal saline-adrenaline injection in colonoscopic polypectomy: prospective randomized study. *Surg Endosc.* 2004;18:990-993.
40. Lee SH, Chung IK, Kim SJ, et al. Comparison of postpolypectomy bleeding between epinephrine and saline submucosal injection for large colon polyps by conventional polypectomy: a prospective randomized, multicenter study. *World J Gastroenterol.* 2007;13:2973-2977.
41. Fyock CJ, Draganov PV. Colonoscopic polypectomy and associated techniques. *World J Gastroenterol.* 2010;16:3630-3637.
42. Di GP, De LL, Calcagno G, Rivellini G, Mandato M, De LB. Detachable snare versus epinephrine injection in the prevention of postpolypectomy bleeding: a randomized and controlled study. *Endoscopy.* 2004;36:860-863.
43. Iishi H, Tatsuta M, Narahara H, Iseki K, Sakai N. Endoscopic resection of large pedunculated colorectal polyps using a detachable snare. *Gastrointest Endosc.* 1996;44:594-597.

44. Paspatis GA, Paraskeva K, Theodoropoulou A, et al. A prospective, randomized comparison of adrenaline injection in combination with detachable snare versus adrenaline injection alone in the prevention of post-polypectomy bleeding in large colonic polyps. *Am J Gastroenterol.* 2006;101:2805.
45. Sobrino-Faya M, Martinez S, Gomez BM, et al. Clips for the prevention and treatment of postpolypectomy bleeding (hemoclips in polypectomy). *Rev Esp Enferm Dig.* 2002;94:457-462.
46. Waye JD. Management of complications of colonoscopic polypectomy. *Gastroenterologist.* 1993;1:158-164.
47. Tolliver KA, Rex DK. Colonoscopic polypectomy. *Gastroenterol Clin North Am.* 2008;37:229-251, ix.
48. Woltjen JA. A retrospective analysis of cecal barotrauma caused by colonoscope air flow and pressure. *Gastrointest Endosc.* 2005;61:37-45.
49. Panteris V, Haringsma J, Kuipers EJ. Colonoscopy perforation rate, mechanisms and outcome: from diagnostic to therapeutic colonoscopy. *Endoscopy.* 2009;41:941-951.
50. Rex DK. Preventing colorectal cancer and cancer mortality with colonoscopy: what we know and what we don't know. *Endoscopy.* 2010;42:320-323.
51. Binmoeller KF, Thonke F, Soehendra N. Endoscopic hemoclip treatment for gastrointestinal bleeding. *Endoscopy.* 1993;25:167-170.
52. Grund KE. Argon plasma coagulation (APC): ballyhoo or breakthrough? *Endoscopy.* 1997;29:196-198.
53. Barker KB, Arnold HL, Fillman EP, Palekar NA, Gering SA, Parker AL. Safety of band ligator use in the small bowel and the colon. *Gastrointest Endosc.* 2005;62:224-227.
54. Witte JT. Band ligation for colonic bleeding: modification of multiband ligating devices for use with a colonoscope. *Gastrointest Endosc.* 2000;52:762-765.
55. Dusold R, Burke K, Carpentier W, Dyck WP. The accuracy of technetium-99m-labeled red cell scintigraphy in localizing gastrointestinal bleeding. *Am J Gastroenterol.* 1994;89:345-348.
56. Loffroy RF, Abualsaud BA, Lin MD, Rao PP. Recent advances in endovascular techniques for management of acute nonvariceal upper gastrointestinal bleeding. *World J Gastrointest Surg.* 2011;3:89-100.
57. Cobb WS, Heniford BT, Sigmon LB, et al. Colonoscopic perforations: incidence, management, and outcomes. *Am Surg.* 2004;70:750-757.
58. Waye JD, Kahn O, Auerbach ME. Complications of colonoscopy and flexible sigmoidoscopy. *Gastrointest Endosc Clin N Am.* 1996;6:343-377.
59. Barbagallo F, Castello G, Latteri S, et al. Successful endoscopic repair of an unusual colonic perforation following polypectomy using an endoclip device. *World J Gastroenterol.* 2007;13:2889-2891.
60. Trecca A, Gaj F, Gagliardi G. Our experience with endoscopic repair of large colonoscopic perforations and review of the literature. *Tech Coloproctol.* 2008;12:315-321
61. Lohsiriwat V. Colonoscopic perforation: incidence, risk factors, management and outcome. *World J Gastroenterol.* 2010;16:425-430.
62. Bleier JI, Moon V, Feingold D, et al. Initial repair of iatrogenic colon perforation using laparoscopic methods. *Surg Endosc.* 2008;22:646-649.

Please visit www.routledge.com/9781617116148 to access additional material.

7

Postcolonoscopy Decision Making
The Guidelines and Beyond

Melissa A. Verrengia, MD and Jeffrey L. Tokar, MD

In the United States, colorectal cancer (CRC) is the third most commonly diagnosed cancer, with approximately 140,000 people receiving this diagnosis every year. CRC is also the second leading cause of cancer-linked deaths. Approximately 50,000 people in whom CRC develops will die of this malignant neoplasm.[1,2] During the past 20 years, both the incidence and mortality rates for CRC in the United States have been declining. This is primarily because of improved CRC screening tests allowing for the early detection and removal of colorectal polyps before they become cancer.[3]

The lifetime risk of CRC is less than 5% in the general population. Among those in whom CRC is diagnosed, 70% would have been considered to have an average risk. The remaining 30% have risk factors that increased their risk for CRC, including a personal or family history of CRC, adenomatous polyps, a personal history of inflammatory bowel disease (IBD), or hereditary genetic syndromes predisposing to CRC (ie, familial adenomatous polyposis [FAP], hereditary nonpolyposis colorectal cancer [HNPCC], or Lynch syndrome).[1]

This chapter will review protocols for screening and surveillance for CRC, including situations not directly addressed in currently available guidelines.

General Screening Recommendations for Average-Risk Individuals

Current CRC screening recommendations for individuals identified as having an average risk are shown in Table 7-1. Most medical societies agree with beginning CRC screening when people are 50 years of age and continuing until they reach the age of approximately 75 to 85 years, although some patients older than 75 will wish to no longer have additional

Adler DG, ed.
Core Concepts in Colonoscopy (pp 81-97).

Table 7-1. Comparison of Average-Risk Screening Colonoscopy Recommendations

SOCIETY/ ORGANIZATION (YEAR)	RECOMMENDATIONS
USMSTF (2012)	• Begin at age 50 • Colonoscopy every 10 years • Flexible sigmoidoscopy, DCBE, or CT colonography every 5 years
ACP (2012)	• Begin at age 50 • Recommends against screening individuals ≥ 75 years or those with substantial comorbidities with < 10-year life expectancy
ACS (2012)	• Begin at age 50 • Flexible sigmoidoscopy every 5 years, colonoscopy every 10 years, DCBE every 5 years, or CT colonography every 5 years
ACG (2009)	• Begin at age 50; continue every 10 years for average risk • Begin at age 45 for African Americans
USPSTF (2008)	• Begin at age 50 to 75 • Recommends against routine screening from ages 76 to 85, but decision should be based on individual patient's comorbidities and results of prior colonoscopies • Stop screening at age 85 years
ASGE (2006)	• Begin at age 50; preferred modality is colonoscopy every 10 years (alternatives: FOBT yearly, flexible sigmoidoscopy every 5 years, or FOBT yearly + flexible sigmoidoscopy every 5 years) • Evidence favors the use of colonoscopy as the primary method for screening, given that a significant portion of proximal advanced neoplasia will not be detected with the use of flexible sigmoidoscopy

Abbreviations: ACG, American College of Gastroenterology; ACP, American College of Physicians; ACS, American Cancer Society; ASGE, American Society for Gastrointestinal Endoscopy; CT, computed tomography; DCBE, double-contrast barium enema; FOBT, fecal occult blood testing; USMSTF, United States Multi-Society Task Force on Colorectal Cancer; USPSTF, United States Preventative Services Task Force.

screening and surveillance examinations. Several modalities (in addition to colonoscopy) have been developed to facilitate the detection of colorectal neoplasia, including indirect stool-based tests (fecal occult blood testing, fecal immunochemical testing, and stool DNA)

Table 7-2. Identifying Individuals at Increased Risk for Colorectal Cancer

- Genetic syndromes predisposing to CRC
  - HNPCC, FAP, and associated variants (attenuated FAP/MYH-associated polyposis, Gardner syndrome, Turcot syndrome)
  - Peutz-Jeghers syndrome, juvenile polyposis syndrome
- Other risks
  - Prior history of CRC or polyps
  - Inflammatory bowel disease
    - Crohn's disease
    - Ulcerative colitis
  - Family history of CRC
  - African American

and tests that identify colorectal neoplasms directly (flexible sigmoidoscopy, double-contrast barium enema [DCBE], computerized tomographic colonography). However, in this chapter we will focus on the use of colonoscopy to detect polyps and CRC.

For average-risk individuals, current CRC screening guidelines from the American Cancer Society (ACS) and the US Multi-Society Task Force on Colorectal Cancer (USMSTF; a collaboration of representatives from the 3 major gastroenterology professional organizations: American College of Gastroenterology [ACG], American Gastroenterological Association [AGA], and American Society for Gastrointestinal Endoscopy [ASGE]) recommend beginning CRC screening when a person reaches the age of 50 years.[4] Among average-risk individuals having CRC screening, 70% to 85% will have no detectable polyps on examination. Assuming the baseline colon examination is complete with an adequate bowel preparation, a repeat colonoscopy can be performed in 10 years.[4]

Colorectal screening and surveillance recommendations for individuals with an above-average risk for CRC are different from the recommendations for average-risk individuals and will be discussed throughout the chapter (Table 7-2).

Screening and Surveillance Recommendations for Individuals With Above-Average Risk for Colorectal Cancer (and Other Unique Clinical Scenarios)

Personal History of Polyps

Polyps will be detected in as many as 30% of average-risk individuals undergoing screening. The most common types of polyps are adenomatous polyps or serrated lesions/

polyps (described in the next section).[5] Those found to have an adenomatous polyp are at increased risk for additional synchronous and metachronous adenomas. For example, the incidence of synchronous adenomas in a person found to have one adenoma is approximately 30% to 50%.[6] Repeat colonoscopy is generally recommended 3 to 5 years after removal of high-risk polyps on baseline colonoscopy. A common problem is that patients with a history of polyps may not be able to provide specific details about their polyp history (eg, "I had a colonoscopy a few years ago in another state, and they said I had a few polyps."). The lack of key data regarding prior colonoscopy findings and histologic results complicates recommendations regarding the timing of follow-up examinations, and optimal surveillance intervals may be less clear in these patients.

Specific recommendations in patients with a history of polyps depend on several factors:

- Pathologic findings for the polyp
  - Adenomatous polyps (tubular, tubulovillous, villous)
  - Serrated lesions (see next section)
- Degree of dysplasia within the polyps
- Number of polyps
- Polyp size
- Adequacy of the bowel preparation at the time of colonoscopy

Personal History of Adenomatous Polyps

Adenomatous Polyps With Only Low-Grade Dysplasia

By definition, adenomatous polyps contain low-grade dysplasia (LGD) and can be characterized further based on histologic characteristics (tubular, villous, tubulovillous) and the number of polyps identified:

- Low-risk adenomas (LRAs) are defined as 1 to 2 tubular adenomas smaller than 10 mm each, with only LGD (Figure 7-1). In this setting, a repeat surveillance colonoscopy is recommended in 5 years.[1,4] Polyps with any villous histologic features have an increased risk of advanced neoplasia during follow-up surveillance intervals (Figure 7-2).[4] Thus, individuals with one or more adenomas that contain villous histologic features (ie, villous or tubulovillous adenomas) without high-grade dysplasia (HGD) should undergo repeat colonoscopy in 3 years. For individuals with 3 to 10 tubular adenomas or more without villous features or HGD, a repeat colonoscopy in 3 years is advised, provided that all adenomatous tissue was completely removed.[1,2,4] If one is uncertain about complete removal, a repeat colonoscopy can be performed in short order (typically 3 months) to evaluate for and remove any residual polyp tissue.
- For individuals with more than 10 polyps, the ACS and USMSTF advise follow-up within 3 years. It is also prudent to consider evaluation for genetic syndromes (eg, variant of FAP) in patients with a significant number of polyps.[2,4]

Adenomatous Polyps With High-Grade Dysplasia

The presence of any adenoma with HGD is an important risk factor for the development of advanced neoplasia and CRC. If one or more adenomas with HGD are found during colonoscopy, a 3-year surveillance interval is recommended, assuming complete polyp removal was achieved.[4] If there is concern about residual polyp tissue, a repeat colonoscopy can be performed within a short period of time.

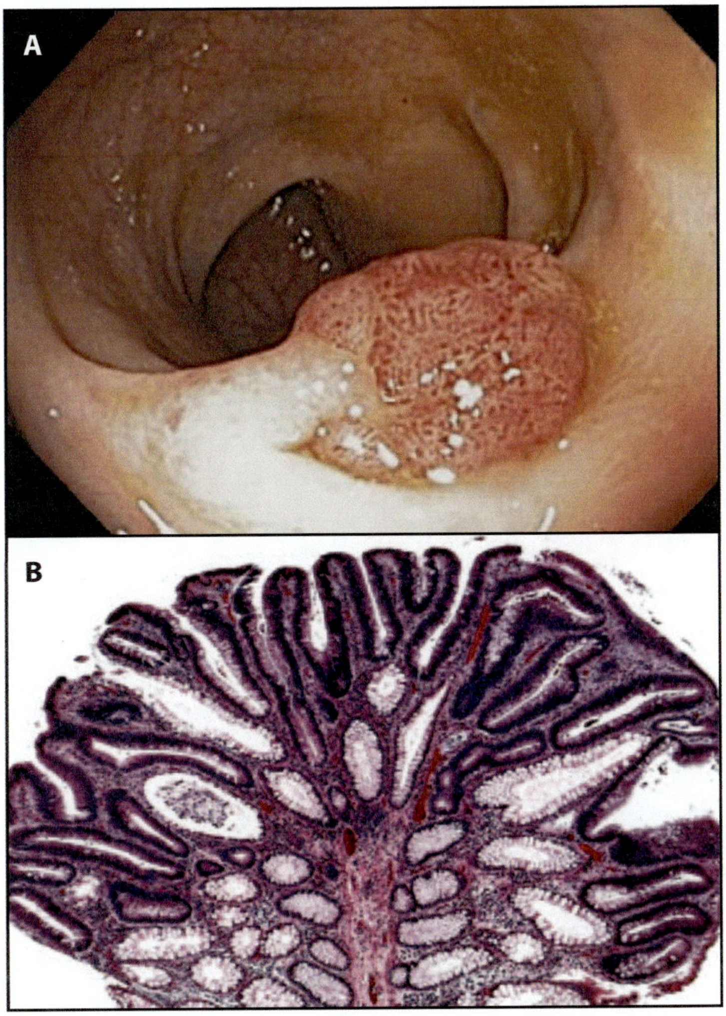

Figure 7-1. Adenoma. (A) A pedunculated polyp seen during colonoscopy. After polypectomy, pathologic examination revealed a tubular adenoma. (Reprinted with permission of Douglas G. Adler, MD.) (B) The colonic adenoma seen here shows dysplasia of the colonic epithelium, characterized by involvement of the full thickness of the mucosa (from the bottom nearest the muscularis mucosae to the surface at the colonic lumen) by enlarged, hyperchromatic, and variably irregular nuclei. This adenoma has a tubular architecture. (Reprinted with permission of Mary Bronner, MD.)

Polyp Size

Individuals with one or more adenomas that are 10 mm or larger also have an increased risk of advanced neoplasia and require a 3-year follow-up colonoscopy once complete resection is achieved.[2,4]

Personal History of Serrated Colorectal Lesions

According to the World Health Organization (WHO), serrated lesions of the large intestine are grouped into 3 categories: hyperplastic polyps (HPs), sessile serrated adenomas/polyps (SSA/Ps) with or without cytological dysplasia, and traditional serrated adenomas (TSAs) (Figure 7-3).[7] These lesions are distinct from adenomatous polyps and are thought to become malignant through an underlying abnormality with CpG island methylation and microsatellite instability rather than through the traditional adenomatous polyposis coli (APC) gene mutation pathway that occurs in adenomatous polyps.[8,9]

HPs show only mild cytologic atypia and are rarely malignant. HPs can be subdivided further based on their histologic characteristics: microvesicular, goblet cell, and mucin-poor types.[10] SSA/Ps and TSAs are considered precancerous lesions.[10] They are difficult to detect on colonoscopy because they are flat or sessile, are of similar color to the

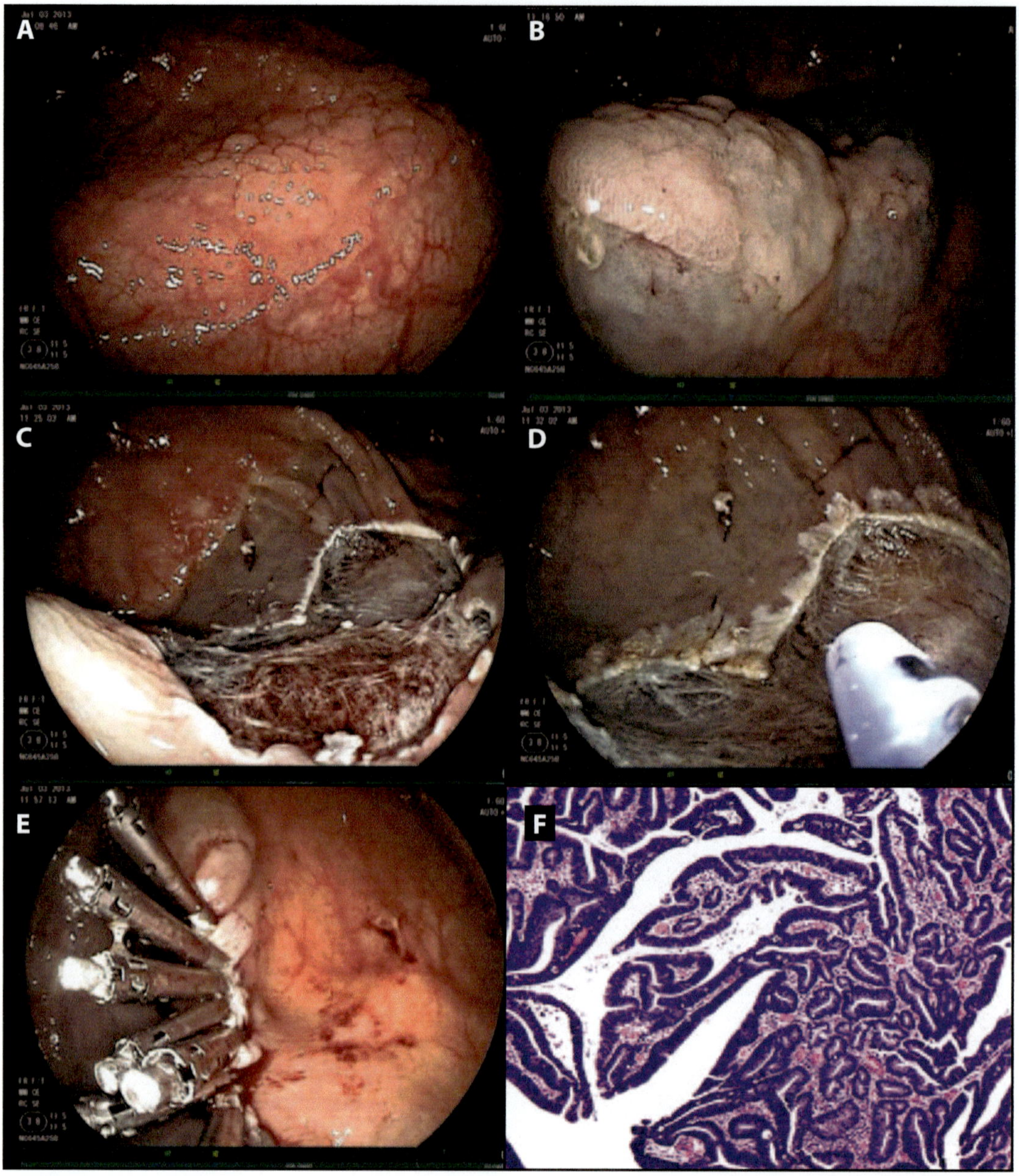

Figure 7-2. Tubulovillous adenoma. (A) A sessile polyp, ultimately shown to be a tubulovillous adenoma, is seen during colonoscopy. (B) Submucosal injection of India ink is performed to lift the lesion and create a submucosal cushion. (C) The appearance of the polypectomy site after hot snare excision. (D) Argon plasma coagulation is used to cauterize the margins of the polypectomy site to fulgurate any remaining polyp tissue. (E) The mucosal defect is closed with several endoscopic clips. (F) This adenomatous polyp demonstrates dysplasia by definition, with enlarged, hyperchromatic, and atypical nuclei that extend onto the surface of the polyp. Its architecture consists of admixed glands or tubules along with fingerlike villous projections. Because of this architectural growth pattern, it is referred to as a *tubulovillous adenoma*. This architectural feature is poorly defined in the literature, ranging from requirements of 25% to 75% for the villous component. It is not defined in any of the published clinical practice guidelines by any of the various gastrointestinal societies and, accordingly, is not applied uniformly by pathologists. However, an increasing villous component predicts an increased risk of adenocarcinoma for an incompletely resected individual adenoma, but it does not reliably predict an increased risk of future neoplasms in the patient's remaining colon. (Reprinted with permission of Mary Bronner, MD.)

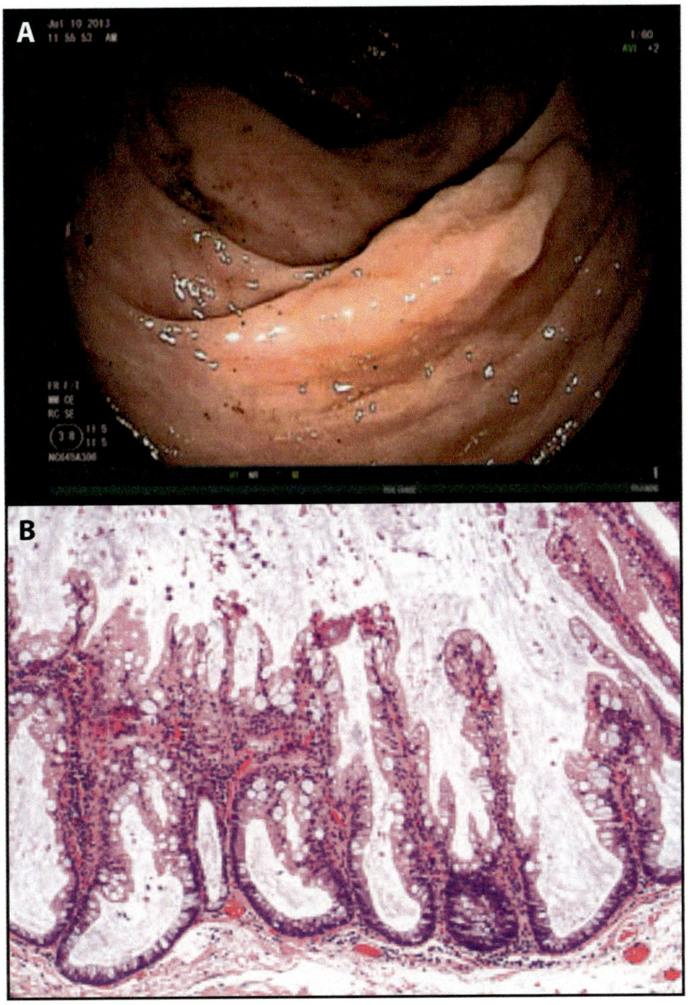

Figure 7-3. Serrated sessile polyp with negative results for dysplasia. (A) Typical appearance of a sessile serrated adenoma in the right colon. (B) This serrated sessile polyp (also known as *serrated sessile adenoma*) shows no evidence of traditional dysplasia and reveals the characteristic (although nondiagnostic) shape. The shape seen here is commonly shared in part by simple HPs, making morphologic characteristics less reproducible as diagnostic criteria. Large polyp size (greater than 1 cm) and right-sided colonic location are more reproducible diagnostic features. The characteristic morphologic features as seen here consist of serrated or jagged/saw-toothed glandular epithelial profiles that extend through the full mucosal thickness of the polyp to also include the polyp base, accompanied by variable cystic dilatation of the serrated glands and lateral extension of the basal-most crypts along the muscularis mucosae (sometimes likened to boot-shaped basal crypts). Serrated sessile polyps also often show a feature that has been termed *crypt dysmaturation*, where the nuclear cytologic characteristics of the basal-most region of the polyp are maintained throughout the full thickness of the polyp to the surface. This is unlike typical HPs that reveal maturation of a more crowded and enlarged basal regenerative nuclear population to normal, very small and bland nuclei as the epithelium extends onto the surface of the polyp. This serrated sessile polyp shows an admixture of dysmaturation and normal maturation, as do most serrated polyps. (Reprinted with permission of Mary Bronner, MD.)

surrounding colonic mucosa, have indiscrete edges, and may contain an associated mucous cap that obscures the underlying polyp and its vascular pattern.[4]

Recommendations for surveillance of individuals with serrated lesions/polyps have been published (Table 7-3).[4,10]

Hyperplastic rectal polyps are relatively common on colonic examination and pose minimal risk of malignancy. If only small (smaller than 10 mm) rectal HPs are found, current guidelines favor a repeat colonoscopy interval of 10 years.[2,4] Size greater than 10 mm and location (proximal to the sigmoid colon) are risk factors that might be associated with a higher risk of CRC.[4] Evidence suggests that an SSA/P with cytologic dysplasia is a more advanced lesion in the progression to cancer compared with an SSA/P without dysplasia.[10]

According to the ACS and USMSTF, an SSA that is 10 mm or larger and an SSA with cytologic dysplasia should be managed as advanced polyps, similar to a high-risk adenoma

Table 7-3. Surveillance Intervals for Serrated Lesions: Expert Consensus Opinion

HISTOLOGIC FINDINGS	SIZE, MM	NUMBER	LOCATION	FOLLOW-UP INTERVAL, Y
HP	< 10	Any	Rectosigmoid	10
HP	≤5	≤3	Proximal to sigmoid	10
HP	Any	≥4	Proximal to sigmoid	5
HP	>5	≥ 1	Proximal to sigmoid	5
SSA/P or TSA	< 10	<3	Any	5
SSA/P or TSA	≥ 10	1	Any	3
SSA/P or TSA	< 10	≥3	Any	3
SSA/P	≥ 10	≥2	Any	1 to 3
SSA/P with dysplasia	Any	Any	Any	1 to 3

(HRA). Serrated lesions smaller than 10 mm that do not display cytologic dysplasia can be managed as LRAs.[4,10] There is currently lack of consensus on identification and grading of dysplasia in TSAs. Thus, the risk of malignancy in TSAs and rate of progression to carcinoma are not known. This may be secondary to a greater degree of heterogeneity in the molecular profile of TSAs compared with SSA/Ps and inconsistencies of diagnostic criteria in these lesions.[10]

Serrated polyposis syndrome (SPS; formerly *hyperplastic polyposis syndrome*) is defined by the WHO as a syndrome with any 1 of the following 3 criteria:

- At least 5 serrated lesions proximal to the sigmoid, with at least 2 lesions larger than 10 mm
- Any number of serrated lesions proximal to the sigmoid colon in an individual with a first-degree relative who has SPS
- More than 20 serrated lesions, of any size, in the colon

The exact risk of CRC in people with SPS is not known. People with SPS in whom CRC develops should have surgery. Extended right hemicolectomy and subtotal colectomy are the most commonly performed operations. Any residual colon or rectum should undergo annual surveillance colonoscopy. Almost 50% of people with SPS have a family history of CRC. Thus, screening colonoscopy at 5-year intervals should be offered to first-degree relatives starting at age 40 years, or 10 years younger than the youngest affected relative.[10] Recommendations regarding surveillance intervals after colonoscopic resection of serrated lesions are based on expert opinion (see Table 7-1).

Incompletely Removed Polyps

Large polyps are sometimes removed in piecemeal fashion because they may be too large for en bloc resection. The ACS and USMSTF advocate a shorter surveillance interval (less than 1 year) if there is any question about how complete resection was, but they acknowledge that there are insufficient data on which to base definitive recommendations.[10] Both the ACS and ASGE recommend repeat examination within 2 to 6 months to remove any remnant polypoid tissue, with 3 months being the most typical time frame.[1,2]

Personal History of Colorectal Cancer

The ASGE recommends that a complete colonoscopy be performed at the time of CRC diagnosis because these individuals have a 3% to 5% risk for development of additional metachronous or synchronous lesions elsewhere within the colon.[1] If a full colonoscopy cannot be completed secondary to an obstructing tumor, a computed tomography colonography or a DCBE can be performed to examine the rest of the colon, although it is known that these studies may be difficult in these people and can miss lesions as well. The ACS recommends that these individuals undergo completion colonoscopy at the time of colorectal surgery or within 3 to 6 months after surgical resection to definitively evaluate the remainder of the colon.[2]

Repeating a colonoscopy on a yearly basis (indefinitely) after resection of nonrectal colon cancer has not been shown to improve survival. Data suggest that the risk for metachronous cancers and polyps appears to be highest during the first 2 years after surgery.[11-13] Thus, the ACS and ASGE recommend a follow-up full colonoscopy 1 year after surgical resection. If adenomatous or high-risk polyps are identified, the examination should be repeated annually until a colonoscopy without adenomas or high-risk lesions is achieved. Subsequently, the examination can be repeated in 3 years. If no adenomas or high-risk lesions are identified, a repeat colonoscopy every 5 years is acceptable.[1,2] The American Society of Clinical Oncology (ASCO) recommends colonoscopy every 3 to 5 years after surgery, whereas the American Society of Colon and Rectal Surgeons (ASCRS) recommends repeat colonoscopy at 3-year intervals.[14,15]

Personal History of Rectal Cancer

According to the ACS and ASCRS, rectal surveillance should be performed every 3 to 6 months for 2 to 3 years after a low anterior resection for rectal cancer.[2,15] The ASCRS also recommends a full colonoscopy at 1 year after diagnosis.[15] In contrast, while acknowledging a 2% to 30% risk of local recurrence within 30 months after the initial resection, the ASGE guidelines emphasize that the optimal surveillance of people with surgically resected rectal cancer is not known.[1] Recent large studies have shown that the combination of preoperative radiation and total mesorectal excision decreases the rate of recurrence in patients with locally advanced rectal cancer to 2.4% within 2 years. For patients with locally advanced disease who did not receive neoadjuvant radiation and those who did not have a total mesorectal excision, the ASCO recommends sigmoidoscopy every 3 to 6 months after surgery for the first 2 to 3 years because their risk of recurrence is approximately 8% within 2 years.[14]

Inflammatory Bowel Disease: Ulcerative Colitis and Crohn's Disease

Individuals with ulcerative colitis (UC) and Crohn's disease are at increased risk for the development of dysplasia and CRC.[1,16] Although IBD accounts for only 1% to 2% of all CRC cases, those with IBD colitis are 6 times more likely to have CRC develop than the general population.[17] Risk factors associated with IBD and CRC include the extent of colitis, longstanding active colitis, disease duration, family history of sporadic CRC, and personal history of primary sclerosing cholangitis (PSC).[1,16] The CRC risk becomes considerable within 7 to 8 years after the onset of pancolitis or 12 to 15 years after the onset of left-sided colitis.[2,17] The goal of CRC surveillance in the population of people with IBD is to detect premalignant changes and prevent invasive cancer. If dysplasia is found in these patients, colectomy is indicated because its presence represents an increased risk factor for progression to CRC.[17]

Ulcerative Colitis

The AGA recommends beginning surveillance colonoscopy in people with pancolitis 8 to 10 years after initial diagnosis and in those with left-sided colitis 15 years after diagnosis. Surveillance should be performed with colonoscopy annually or biannually.[18,19] Two to 4 random mucosal biopsies should be taken every 10 cm along the length of the colon or in each segment of the colon and rectum (ie, cecum, ascending colon, hepatic flexure, transverse colon, splenic flexure, descending colon, sigmoid colon, and rectum, which also roughly corresponds to every 10 cm). Special attention is paid to the rectosigmoid colon because there is an increased frequency of CRC in this area. Some experts advocate 4-quadrant random biopsies every 5 cm, with particular attention paid to suspicious areas, but this is not widely performed.[17]

The ACG recommends annual colonoscopy with multiple mucosal biopsies to evaluate for dysplasia beginning 8 to 10 years after diagnosis in patients who are considered surgical candidates, including those with left-sided colitis, for whom there are insufficient data to recommend alternative surveillance recommendations. They do not specify whether surveillance can begin later in those with only left-sided disease.[20] If any grade of dysplasia is present, colectomy is recommended (Figure 7-4). Repeat surveillance colonoscopies at shorter intervals are recommended for patients whose biopsy specimens have indefinite findings for dysplasia.[21]

The ASGE, which has issued recommendations similar to those from the ACG and AGA, also recommends colonoscopic surveillance after 8 years for patients with pancolitis and 15 years for those with left-sided colitis, with 4 biopsies every 10 cm from cecum to rectum and targeted biopsies of any suspect areas, advocating an annual to semiannual interval (every 2 years). However, the ASGE differs in its recommendations concerning patients with IBD with LGD. If findings of LGD are confirmed by an expert pathologist, the ASGE guidelines allow for consideration of frequent colonoscopic surveillance (every 3 to 6 months) as an alternative to colectomy, particularly for patients in whom colectomy is not feasible or is unacceptable. If there is any evidence of HGD—or any degree of dysplasia associated with an endoscopically visible lesion or mass—or evidence of carcinoma, colectomy is advised. Surveillance colonoscopy is not indicated in patients who have ulcerative proctitis.[1]

The association of PSC with UC has been known for many years. The cumulative CRC risk in these people has been reported to be 33% at 20 years and 40% at 30 years from the time of UC diagnosis. Because the CRC risk in this patient population is high,

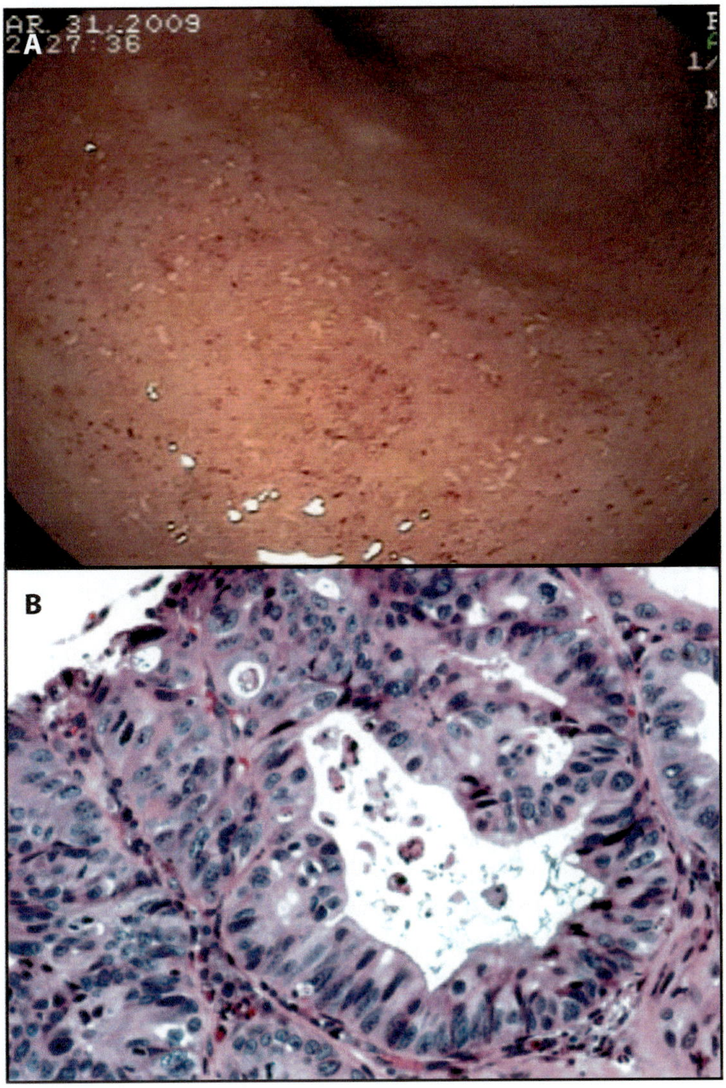

Figure 7-4. UC with HGD. (A) Mucosal image in a patient with UC obtained during surveillance colonoscopy. Note the loss of haustral folds and normal vascular pattern. There are innumerable small mucosal ulcerations as well. (B) This biopsy specimen, taken from a patient with UC, illustrates the diagnostic cytoarchitectural features of HGD. These include the continuous variable criteria without precise cutoffs from LGD, namely nuclear enlargement, hyperchromasia, and pleomorphism, along with the more dichotomous criterion (which is therefore more objective), namely loss of nuclear polarity. This latter feature refers to loss of a perpendicular orientation of the long axis of the nucleus relative to the basal lamina so that the nuclei instead become more rounded and disordered relative to the basal lamina and to each other. In addition to these cytologic features, this biopsy specimen shows significant glandular crowding, cribriform change (single glandular structure with multiple lumens), and dilated glands with necrotic luminal debris, all architectural patterns highly characteristic of HGD. (Reprinted with permission of Mary Bronner, MD.)

annual colonoscopic surveillance from the time of PSC diagnosis has been advised but is not universally accepted or practiced.[17]

Crohn's Disease

People with Crohn's disease with extensive disease involving more than one-third of the colon appear to have an increased risk of CRC, similar to that of people with UC. Because detection of CRC in Crohn's disease can be delayed inadvertently and be associated with a worse prognosis, surveillance colonoscopy has been recommended in these people every 1 to 2 years with systematic biopsies to detect dysplasia, similar to recommendations for people with UC.[1]

Genetic Syndromes Associated With Colorectal Cancer

Familial Adenomatous Polyposis

FAP is defined as an autosomal-dominant syndrome occurring secondary to a germline mutation in the APC gene (a tumor suppressor). FAP is characterized by the development of hundreds to thousands of colonic adenomas by the time a person reaches early adolescence. These individuals have a nearly 100% risk for development of CRC by age 40 to 50 years if the colon is not removed.[1] Additionally, the risk of gastroduodenal cancer developing in people with FAP with gastroduodenal polyposis is approximately 7%.[22] Screening for upper gastrointestinal neoplasia in these people is beyond the scope of this chapter but is usually performed as well.

FAP accounts for less than 1% of the total number of people with CRC in the United States. Genetic testing is available for individuals and family members believed to be at risk for FAP. For those with a detectable APC mutation, genetic testing of at-risk family members may be appropriate. In such cases, absence of the familial APC gene mutation in a family member suggests FAP will not develop. However, in settings where genetic testing is not available or is deemed to be inappropriate or out of financial reach, endoscopic screening for the development of polyposis is recommended.

Average patient age when polyps begin to form is 15 years. Thus, the ACS and ASGE recommend initiating screening (with annual flexible sigmoidoscopy) for at-risk individuals between ages 10 to 12 years and consideration of prophylactic colectomy if multiple polyps are found.[1,2] If no polyps are detected, annual flexible sigmoidoscopy should continue until the patient is 40 years of age, then every 3 to 4 years thereafter.[1]

Although relatives of people with FAP with normal genetic test results are assumed not to have FAP, some experts advocate performing flexible sigmoidoscopy every 7 to 10 years until these people reach the age of 40 years, then colonoscopy every 5 years thereafter to account for potential errors in genetic testing.[1] If a mutation is not identified in a family with FAP, annual flexible sigmoidoscopy can be offered to at-risk family members from age 13 to 15 years until age 30. Then the interval can increase to every 3 to 4 years until they reach the age of 60. Surgery should be strongly recommended for all people with FAP before they reach the age of 25.[22]

For people with known FAP or those at risk for FAP because of family history, the ACG recommends yearly flexible sigmoidoscopy or colonoscopy until such time as colectomy is deemed by the physician and patient to be the best treatment. If a patient with FAP undergoes subtotal colectomy with ileoanal anastomosis, the risk for cancer in the retained rectum is 12% to 29%. Thus, surveillance with flexible sigmoidoscopy every 6 to 12 months is advisable.[23] After restorative proctocolectomy, lifelong annual surveillance also is necessary for the anorectal cuff.[22]

Hereditary Nonpolyposis Colorectal Cancer

HNPCC (also known as *Lynch syndrome*) is an autosomal-dominant, familial form of CRC caused by mutations in DNA mismatch repair genes. The syndrome accounts for approximately 2% to 3% of all CRCs. People with HNPCC also have increased risk for other cancers, including endometrial, stomach, ovarian, biliary tract, pancreatic, kidney, ureteral, and brain (usually glioblastoma multiforme). The lifetime risk for CRC in these individuals is approximately 70% to 80%, and right-sided colon cancers are unusually prevalent.[24] HNPCC should be suspected in people with one or more of the Revised Bethesda Criteria[25]:

- CRC diagnosed in a patient who is younger than 50 years
- Presence of synchronous or metachronous CRC and other HNPCC syndrome-associated tumors (listed previously), regardless of age
- CRC with high microsatellite instability diagnosed in a patient younger than 60 years
- CRC diagnosed in an individual with 1 or more first-degree relatives with an HNPCC-associated tumor, with one of the cancers being diagnosed when the person is younger than 50 years
- CRC diagnosed in 2 or more first- or second-degree relatives with an HNPCC-associated tumor (regardless of age)

The ACS, ACG, and ASGE recommend beginning screening at-risk individuals at age 20 to 25 years or 10 years earlier than the age at which the youngest affected family member received a diagnosis, using colonoscopy every 1 to 2 years.[1,2,23] When a person reaches 40 years of age, annual colonoscopy is advised. Screening recommendations for the other HNPCC-associated cancers is beyond the scope of this chapter but should be discussed with at-risk individuals.

Peutz-Jeghers Syndrome

Peutz-Jeghers syndrome (PJS) is a rare autosomal-dominant syndrome with high penetrance associated with defects in a serine threonine kinase (STK11) in most patients.[26] Those with PJS have multiple hamartomatous polyps of the small intestine, colon, and rectum develop in association with mucocutaneous pigmentation. Hamartomatous polyps are most common in the small intestine (65% to 95% of patients) but also arise in the colon (60%) and stomach (50%), with cumulative cancer risks in patients from ages 15 to 64 of 13%, 39%, and 29%, respectively. Those with PJS are also at significant risk of other extraintestinal malignant tumors (eg, breast, pancreas, ovary, lung, uterus, or cervix).[27] Hamartomas, particularly when large, can be associated with bleeding, bowel obstruction, and a low rate of malignant transformation (3%). Many experts recommend removal of only polyps larger than 1 cm because of a greater potential for complications. People with PJS are at risk for extraintestinal malignant neoplasms, including cancers of the pancreas, liver, breast, ovaries, uterus, lungs, and testes. The cumulative lifetime cancer risk by the time someone reaches the age of 70 years is approximately 85%. By age 70 years, the risk for all gastrointestinal cancers (eg, colon and rectum, pancreas, and small bowel) is approximately 57%, with a lifetime CRC risk of 10% to 20%.[22] Current screening recommendations include baseline upper endoscopy, colonoscopy or flexible sigmoidoscopy with barium enema, and small-bowel imaging (eg, video capsule endoscopy) in patients aged 8 years. If polyps are detected, repeat examination is advisable at 3-year intervals until the patient is 50 years of age. If no polyps are detected on baseline examinations, then 3-year-interval surveillance can resume when the patient reaches the age of 18 years until 50 years, or earlier if symptoms arise. At age 50, colonoscopy intervals should increase to every 1 to 2 years because of the rapid increase in cancer risk.

Juvenile Polyposis Syndrome

Juvenile polyposis syndrome is defined by the presence of multiple typical hamartomatous polyps of the colon and rectum. This syndrome usually manifests itself during childhood. The lifetime risk of CRC is between 10% and 38%, and colonoscopic surveillance of asymptomatic individuals is recommended starting between the ages of 15 and 18 years, followed by colonoscopy every 1 to 2 years until the age of 70 years. Prophylactic colectomy should be discussed.[22]

Family History

Individuals with a first-degree relative with CRC are at increased risk for colonic neoplasia. Similarly, individuals with a first-degree relative with large adenomas may have a greater risk for CRC and large adenomas, particularly if the family member was younger than 60 years at diagnosis, was male, or had a large adenoma in the left-sided colorectum.[28]

The most cost-effective approach for family members remains to be defined. The joint ACS and USMSTF recommendations for relatives who do not meet criteria for HNPCC are as follows: individuals with CRC or adenomatous polyps in a first-degree relative younger than 60 years or 2 or more first-degree relatives at any age should have colonoscopy every 5 years beginning at age 40 (or 10 years earlier than the youngest family member was at diagnosis). For individuals with a first-degree relative who was age 60 years or older at diagnosis or with 2 second-degree relatives with CRC, they recommend an initial screening examination when the patient is at an early age (40 years) but continuing at intervals that are used for average-risk individuals.[29,30] Patients with a single second- or third-degree relative with CRC should adhere to average-risk screening recommendations.[1]

In 2009, the ACG published separate but similar recommendations advocating the following for first-degree relatives with CRC or advanced adenomas (defined as villous elements on histologic examination, larger than 10 mm in size, presence of HGD): individuals with a single first-degree relative with CRC or advanced adenoma at age 60 years or older should be offered screening at the same age and intervals as average-risk individuals, whereas persons with 2 or more first-degree relatives diagnosed with CRC or advanced adenoma at any age, or a single first-degree relative diagnosed before age 60, should have screening every 5 years beginning at age 40 years or 10 years earlier than the age at which the youngest affected family member received a diagnosis.[23]

Individuals with normal results on a baseline colonoscopic examination who have a first-degree relative with CRC or HRA younger than 60 years at the time of diagnosis should undergo repeat colonoscopy at 5-year intervals. This is because of an increased lifetime risk of CRC (2 to 3 times higher) than the general population. However, if the first-degree relative was 60 years or older at the time of diagnosis, repeat colonoscopy should continue at 10-year intervals.[4,5]

A major complicating factor is that many individuals will have a poor or nonexistent knowledge and understanding of the medical history of their family members. The person may be completely unaware of a family history of polyps and/or CRC, or he or she may have only a partial family history. Similarly, people who are adopted may have no way to access information about the medical history of their blood relatives. In these people, if there is any concern about possible family members with a history of CRC or an advanced adenoma and details cannot be obtained, the clinician usually makes a best-guess decision about the timing and frequency of future colonoscopic examinations that can be based on the patient's overall personal history and available family history.

Ethnicity

African Americans have the highest incidence of CRC, and there are data suggesting that African Americans are at risk for development of CRC at younger ages compared with other racial or ethnic groups. As such, the current guidelines from the American College of Physicians (ACP) recommend initiating CRC screening when African Americans reach the age of 40, whereas the ACG and ASGE recommend screening of African Americans beginning at age 45.[1,4,31]

Recommendations for Patients With Inadequate Bowel Preparation or Incomplete Colonoscopy

Inadequate bowel preparation is defined as the inability to visualize polyps that are 5 mm or larger. A recent study reported that among average-risk individuals undergoing repeat colonoscopy for inadequate bowel preparation, adenomas and high-risk lesions were frequently detected, suggesting that they were missed on the initial colonoscopy.[32] The ACS and USMSTF recommend that, in most cases of inadequate bowel preparation, the examination should be repeated within 1 year. However, if the bowel preparation was adequate to detect lesions larger than 5 mm and if only small (less than 10 mm) tubular adenomas are detected, a follow-up colonoscopy at 5 years may be considered.[4] The ASGE recommendations advocate for a short-interval follow-up colonoscopy if bowel preparation is poor (or, similarly, if the examination was not completed to the cecum) but do not provide specific timing recommendations.[1]

In some cases, the bowel preparation is believed to be adequate overall for a colonoscopy to the cecum but less than optimal compared with an ideal preparation. In these situations, the physician must make a decision regarding repeating the examination in the immediate future (it is hoped with a better bowel preparation) or asking the patient to return for a subsequent examination on a shortened time frame (eg, 3 years).

Recommendations for Individuals at Advanced Ages

The WHO defines the elderly as individuals 65 years or older. An increased incidence of CRC is seen in elderly people compared with younger people. However, the gain in life expectancy from the use of screening colonoscopy diminishes with increasing age and is significantly less for individuals older than 80 years.[33] The United States Preventative Services Task Force recommends against routine CRC screening in people older than 75 years and advocates against all screening in people older than 85 because the procedure risk exceeds the potential benefit. The ACP recommends that clinicians stop screening for CRC in adults older than the age of 75 years or in adults with a life expectancy of less than 10 years, although this can be somewhat difficult to gauge in reality.[31] The ACS and USMSTF do not recommend an absolute age at which to discontinue screening, advising that decisions to continue screening or surveillance in elderly people should be based on the assessment of benefit, risk, and comorbidities in an individual patient.[4] Ultimately, the decision to continue screening and surveillance examinations in patients of advanced age remains a balance between age, life expectancy, comorbid medical conditions, and risk of colonoscopy. A frank discussion with the patient regarding future colonoscopy examinations is often helpful in making these decisions because some people will feel strongly about continuing CRC screening and surveillance, whereas others will have a lower threshold to discontinue such tests. Healthy elderly patients who wish to continue having screening colonoscopy should not necessarily be discouraged.

Conclusion

Guidelines for CRC screening and surveillance continue to evolve as we gain greater understanding of the natural history of colorectal neoplasms, risk factors for CRC, and performance characteristics of various existing and emerging diagnostic modalities. The information provided in this chapter is a summary of currently available recommendations and is intended to serve as a guide for clinicians involved in making screening or surveillance recommendations for patients and their family members.

References

1. Davila RE, Rajan E, Baron TH, et al. ASGE guideline: colorectal cancer screening and surveillance. *Gastrointest Endosc.* 2006;63(4):546-557.
2. American Cancer Society. Colorectal cancer facts and figures, 2011-2013. http://www.cancer.org/acs/groups/content/@epidemiologysurveilance/documents/document/acspc-028323.pdf. Accessed February 1, 2013.
3. Centers for Disease Control and Prevention. Vital signs: colorectal cancer screening, incidence, and mortality—United States, 2002-2010. *MMWR Morb Mortal Wkly Rep.* 2011;60(26):884-889.
4. Lieberman DA, Rex DK, Winawer SJ, et al. Guidelines for colonoscopy surveillance after screening and polypectomy: a consensus update by the US Multi-Society Task Force on Colorectal Cancer. *Gastroenterology.* 2012;143(3):844-857.
5. Rudy DR, Zdon MJ. Update on colorectal cancer. *Am Fam Physician.* 2000;61(6):1759-1770, 1773-1774.
6. Bond JH. Polyp guideline: diagnosis, treatment, and surveillance for patients with colorectal polyps. Practice Parameters Committee of the American College of Gastroenterology. *Am J Gastroenterol.* 2000;95(11):3053-3063.
7. Snover D, Ahnen D, Burt R, et al. *Serrated Polyps of the Colon and Rectum and Serrated ("Hyperplastic") Polyposis.* Vol. 4. Berlin, Germany: Springer-Verlag; 2010.
8. Noffsinger AE. Serrated polyps and colorectal cancer: new pathway to malignancy. *Ann Rev Pathol.* 2009;4:343-364.
9. Sweetser S, Smyrk T, Sinicrope F. Serrated colon polyps as precursors to colorectal cancer. *Clin Gastroenterol Hepatol.* 2013;11(7):760-767.
10. Rex DK, Ahnen DJ, Baron JA, et al. Serrated lesions of the colorectum: review and recommendations from an expert panel. *Am J Gastroenterol.* 2012;107(9):1315-1329.
11. Makela JT, Laitinen SO, Kairaluoma MI. Five-year follow-up after radical surgery for colorectal cancer. Results of a prospective randomized trial. *Arch Surg.* 1995;130(10):1062-1067.
12. Ohlsson B, Breland U, Ekberg H, Graffner H, Tranberg KG. Follow-up after curative surgery for colorectal carcinoma. Randomized comparison with no follow-up. *Dis Colon Rectum.* 1995;38(6):619-626.
13. Schoemaker D, Black R, Giles L, Toouli J. Yearly colonoscopy, liver CT, and chest radiography do not influence 5-year survival of colorectal cancer patients. *Gastroenterology.* 1998;114(1):7-14.
14. Benson AB III, Desch CE, Flynn PJ, et al. 2000 update of American Society of Clinical Oncology colorectal cancer surveillance guidelines. *J Clin Oncol.* 2000;18(20):3586-3588.
15. Anthony T, Simmang C, Hyman N, et al. Practice parameters for the surveillance and follow-up of patients with colon and rectal cancer. *Dis Colon Rectum.* 2004;47(6):807-817.
16. Freeman HJ. Colorectal cancer risk in Crohn's disease. *World J Gastroenterol.* 2008;14(12):1810-1811.

17. Mattar MC, Lough D, Pishvaian MJ, Charabaty A. Current management of inflammatory bowel disease and colorectal cancer. *Gastrointest Cancer Res.* 2011;4(2):53-61.
18. Farraye FA, Odze RD, Eaden J, et al. AGA medical position statement on the diagnosis and management of colorectal neoplasia in inflammatory bowel disease. *Gastroenterology.* 2010;138(2):738-745.
19. Farraye FA, Odze RD, Eaden J, Itzkowitz SH. AGA technical review on the diagnosis and management of colorectal neoplasia in inflammatory bowel disease. *Gastroenterology.* 2010;138(2):746-774, 774.e1-e4.
20. Kornbluth A, Sachar DB. Ulcerative colitis practice guidelines in adults: American College of Gastroenterology, Practice Parameters Committee. *Am J Gastroenterol.* 2010;105(3):501-523.
21. Kornbluth A, Sachar DB. Ulcerative colitis practice guidelines in adults. American College of Gastroenterology, Practice Parameters Committee. *Am J Gastroenterol.* 1997;92(2):204-211.
22. Katballe N, Christensen M, Wikman FP, Orntoft TF, Laurberg S. Frequency of hereditary non-polyposis colorectal cancer in Danish colorectal cancer patients. *Gut.* 2002;50(1):43-51.
23. Rex D, Johnson D, Anderson J, Schoenfeld P, Burke C, Inadomi J. American College of Gastroenterology guidelines for colorectal cancer screening 2008. *Am J Gastroenterol.* 2009;104:739-750.
24. Quehenberger F, Vasen HF, van Houwelingen HC. Risk of colorectal and endometrial cancer for carriers of mutations of the hMLH1 and hMSH2 gene: correction for ascertainment. *J Med Genet.* 2005;42(6):491-496.
25. Umar A, Boland CR, Terdiman JP, et al. Revised Bethesda guidelines for hereditary nonpolyposis colorectal cancer (Lynch syndrome) and microsatellite instability. *J Natl Cancer Inst.* 2004;96(4):261-268.
26. Jenne DE, Reimann H, Nezu J, et al. Peutz-Jeghers syndrome is caused by mutations in a novel serine threonine kinase. *Nat Genet.* 1998;18(1):38-43.
27. Giardiello FM, Brensinger JD, Tersmette AC, et al. Very high risk of cancer in familial Peutz-Jeghers syndrome. *Gastroenterology.* 2000;119(6):1447-1453.
28. Cottet V, Pariente A, Nalet B, et al. Colonoscopic screening of first-degree relatives of patients with large adenomas: increased risk of colorectal tumors. *Gastroenterology.* 2007;133(4):1086-1092.
29. Levin B, Lieberman DA, McFarland B, et al. Screening and surveillance for the early detection of colorectal cancer and adenomatous polyps, 2008: a joint guideline from the American Cancer Society, the US Multi-Society Task Force on Colorectal Cancer, and the American College of Radiology. *CA Cancer J Clin.* 2008;58(3):130-160.
30. Levin B, Lieberman DA, McFarland B, et al. Screening and surveillance for the early detection of colorectal cancer and adenomatous polyps, 2008: a joint guideline from the American Cancer Society, the US Multi-Society Task Force on Colorectal Cancer, and the American College of Radiology. *Gastroenterology.* 2008;134(5):1570-1595.
31. Qaseem A, Denberg TD, Hopkins RH Jr, et al. Screening for colorectal cancer: a guidance statement from the American College of Physicians. *Ann Intern Med.* 2012;156(5):378-386.
32. Chokshi RV, Hovis CE, Hollander T, Early DS, Wang JS. Prevalence of missed adenomas in patients with inadequate bowel preparation on screening colonoscopy. *Gastrointest Endosc.* 2012;75(6):1197-1203.
33. Day LW, Walter LC, Velayos F. Colorectal cancer screening and surveillance in the elderly patient. *Am J Gastroenterol.* 2011;106(7):1197-1206.

8

Colonoscopy Perforations
How to Avoid Them and What to Do if They Happen

Louis M. Wong Kee Song, MD and Todd H. Baron, MD

Perforation as a result of colonoscopy is a rare but potentially life-threatening adverse event. The perforation rates for diagnostic procedures vary from 0.01% to 0.8% and are as high as 5% for therapeutic procedures, such as endoscopic submucosal dissection (ESD).[1,2] Risk factors for colonoscopic perforation include, but are not limited to, advanced age, severe comorbid medical illnesses, female sex, diverticulosis, previous abdominopelvic surgery, colonic obstruction and pseudoobstruction as an indication, and therapeutic interventions.[2,3]

Mechanisms of Injury

Perforations that occur during diagnostic colonoscopy tend to be large and are often caused by direct mechanical injury. This includes stretching of the bowel wall during advancement of the endoscope through formation of a loop and during retroflexion. The other mechanism of injury is barotrauma due to excessive air insufflation, especially in the setting of obstruction with a *closed-loop phenomenon*. The rectosigmoid colon is a vulnerable area because diverticular disease is often present in this segment of the colon, and the sigmoid colon may be redundant, narrowed, angulated, and/or fixated because of pelvic adhesions.[4] Such adhesions are common after pelvic surgery, including hysterectomy.

Therapeutic procedures such as dilation, stent placement, and resection of large polyps can result in perforation. Perforations due to polypectomy are caused most often by thermal injury that occurs during hot-snare polypectomy, bipolar coagulation, and argon plasma coagulation (APC). Therapy-related perforations are usually smaller than those caused by direct mechanical injury because they occur at targeted sites of intervention rather than

Adler DG, ed.
Core Concepts in Colonoscopy (pp 99-112).

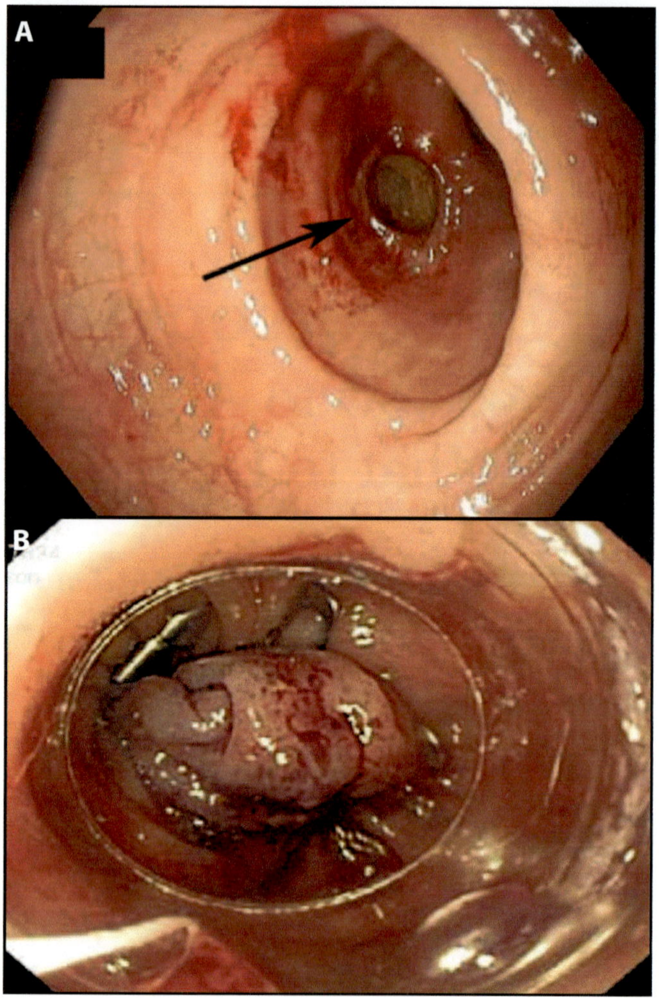

Figure 8-1. (A) Colonoscopic perforation of a sigmoid diverticulum (B) closed with an over-the-scope clip.

along broad expanses of colon wall and thus are more amenable to endoscopic closure. This is supported by a study in which the mean perforation diameter after diagnostic procedures was 19.3 mm compared with 5.8 mm for therapeutic procedures.[5] In another study, 88% of perforations that occurred during diagnostic colonoscopy required laparotomy compared with only 9% of perforations related to therapeutic colonoscopy.[6]

Prevention of Colonoscopic Perforations

The use of appropriate technique and accessories can minimize the risk for colonoscopic perforation. First, blind advancement of the colonoscope without visualization of the lumen should be avoided, particularly in the presence of dense diverticular disease where the tip of the endoscope can easily impact and perforate a diverticulum (Figure 8-1). Second, forceful advancement should be avoided when resistance is encountered, and only experienced proceduralists should use the slide-by technique. When a patient verbalizes or reacts to pain, one should be especially concerned about formation of a loop. However, patient feedback is lost when anesthesia support and/or deep sedation is used (ie, the patient cannot feel pain and thus cry out, so the endoscopist is not alerted to a potential problem). Prevention of loop formation and reduction of loops upon recognition are also important maneuvers to minimize bowel-stretch injury.

In patients with dense colonic diverticula, one must be especially cautious. Diverticula can be negotiated carefully with patience, gentle advancement, and gentle insufflation of air or carbon dioxide or by distending the lumen with water insufflation instead of gas. In patients with anticipated colonic difficulties (eg, known diverticulosis and/or a history of pelvic surgery), use of a thinner and more flexible endoscope, such as a pediatric colonoscope or even an upper endoscope, can be particularly helpful. One should have a low threshold for switching from an adult to a pediatric colonoscope when the left colon cannot be negotiated easily. In extreme cases of angulation or redundancy of the sigmoid colon, balloon-assisted endoscopy can be useful because of the small diameter and increased flexibility of the enteroscope and capability of performing efficient endoscope-reduction maneuvers.

Avoidance of excessive air insufflation, especially in the setting of a colonic obstruction or pseudo-obstruction, can prevent barotrauma-related perforation. In this circumstance, it is preferable to insufflate with carbon dioxide, which is absorbed rapidly relative to air. Alternatively, water insufflation also can reduce this risk.

The risk of APC-induced colonic perforation can be minimized by avoiding probe-tissue contact and limiting the duration of application to 1- to 2-second pulses. It is important to avoid overdistension of the lumen, particularly in the cecum, because the thinner colonic wall found in the proximal colon is more prone to transmural injury during APC application. Similarly, light tissue pressure should be used when contact thermal probes, such as with bipolar coagulation, are used. The creation of a submucosal fluid cushion provides some protection for the underlying muscularis propria and should be used during endoscopic mucosal resection (EMR) of flat or large lesions in the colon, although perforation can occur even after creation of a submucosal fluid cushion.

Diagnosis of Colonoscopic Perforations

Intraprocedural perforation is obvious when a mural tear occurs with resultant direct endoscopic visualization of intra-abdominal organs or serosal fat (Figure 8-2). Excessive abdominal distention, especially in the setting of pain and persistence of distension despite air suction and loop reduction, should alert the endoscopist to the possibility of a perforation. The development of tension pneumoperitoneum, manifested by a tense abdomen with respiratory compromise and hypotension, requires emergent placement of a large-bore needle catheter to prevent cardiovascular collapse.[7] Intraprocedural perforation may not be obvious and can be missed endoscopically when the mural defect is small in the absence of overt physical signs and symptoms.

Recently, a potential indication of full-thickness bowel wall resection with resulting perforation, called the *target sign*, has been described.[8] This is an endoscopic marker of injury to the muscularis propria and is seen best after dye-assisted EMR. A mirror image of the target sign also can be seen on the underside of the resected polyp. If recognized at endoscopy, the defect in the bowel wall should be closed (Figure 8-3).

After the procedure, a perforation should be considered and evaluated appropriately when a patient reports persistent abdominal pain. An upright radiograph of the lower

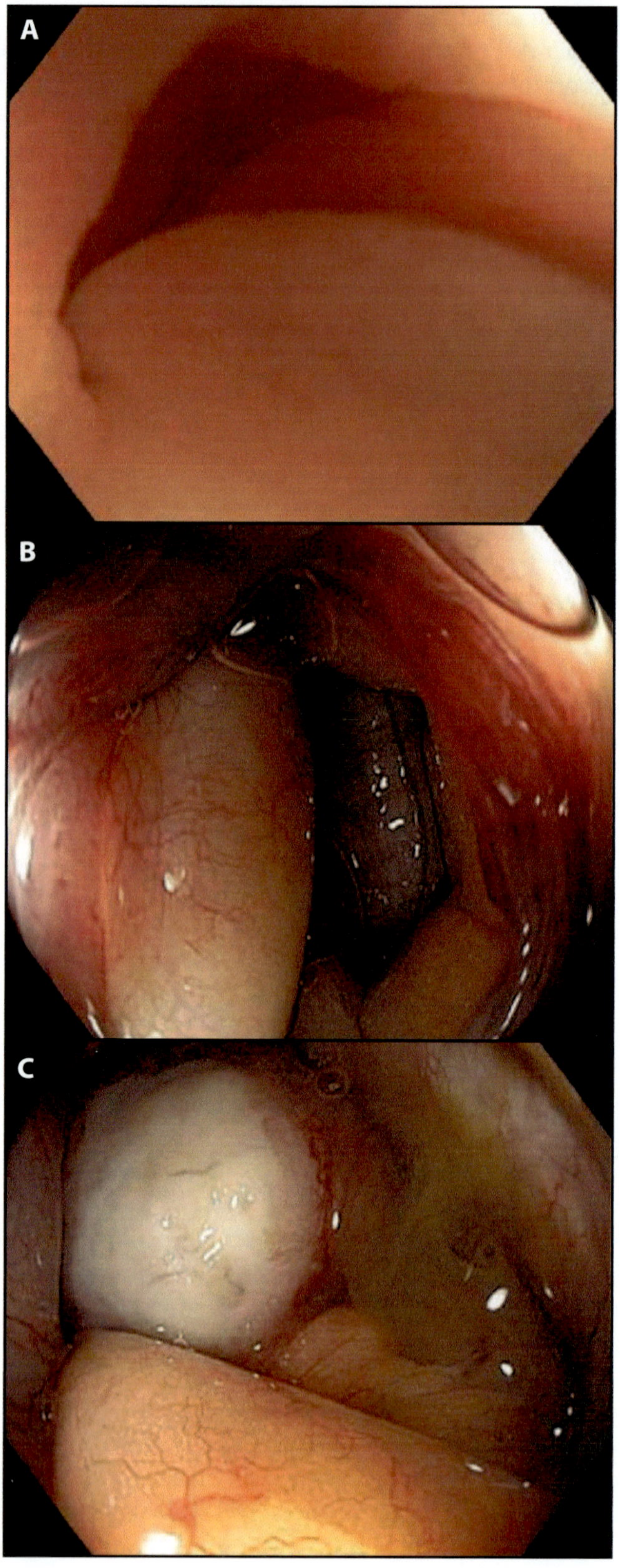

Figure 8-2. (A) Difficult colonoscope passage through a narrowed and angulated sigmoid colon, resulting in (B) a perforation and large gaping tear, with visualization of (C) serosal fat and intra-abdominal organs.

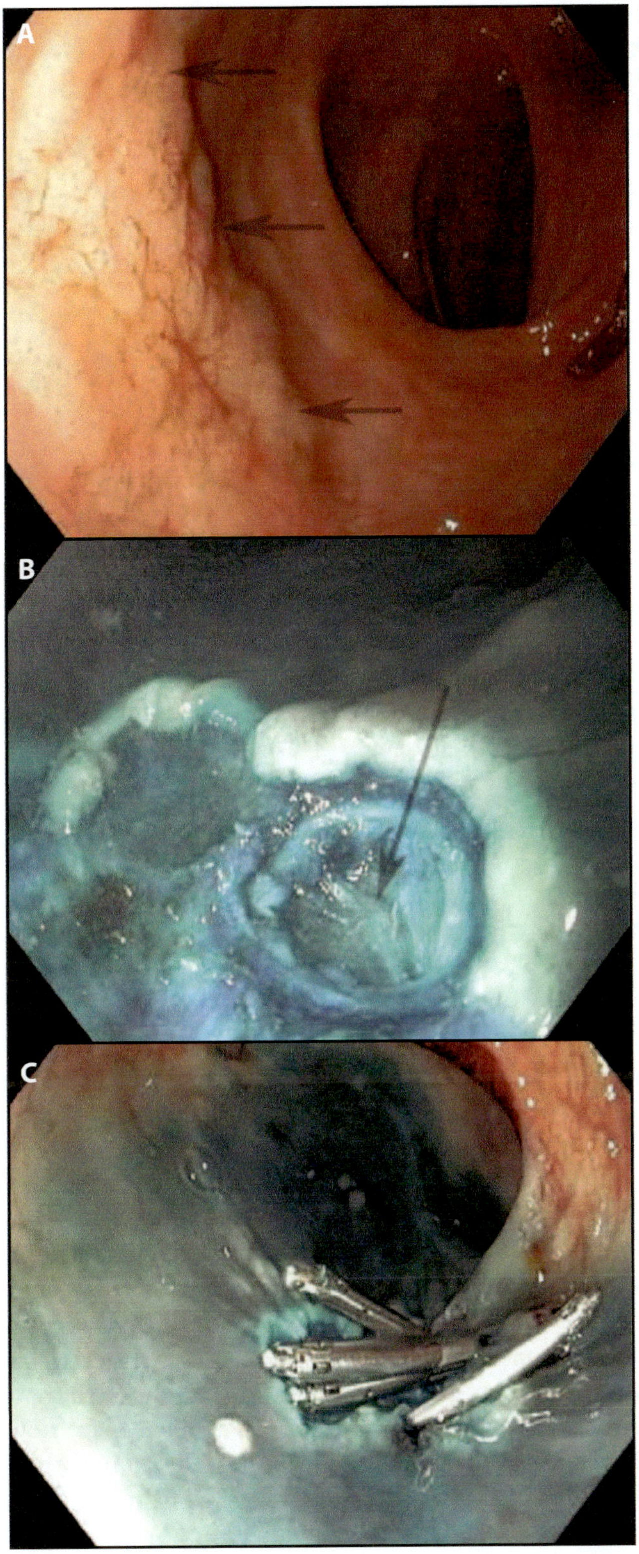

Figure 8-3. (A) Piecemeal snare resection of a large sessile polyp resulting in (B) muscularis propria injury and the target sign, which was (C) closed promptly with endoscopic clips.

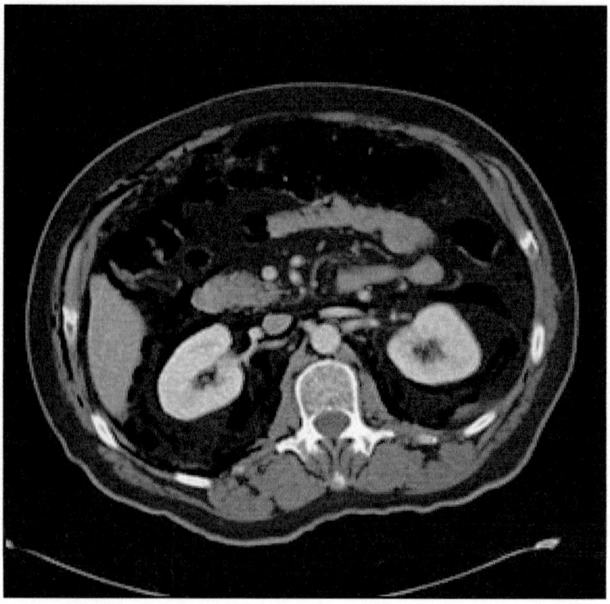

Figure 8-4. Abdominal CT scan showing a moderate amount of retroperitoneal and intraperitoneal air after cecal perforation from polypectomy.

chest and upper abdomen may reveal free air. However, the absence of free air under the diaphragm on plain abdominal radiographs does not rule out perforation. An abdominal computed tomography (CT) scan is more sensitive at detecting extraluminal (especially retroperitoneal) air and should be performed when there is a high index of suspicion for perforation (Figure 8-4).

Management of Colonoscopic Perforations

Endoscopic Closure Versus Operative Repair

The decision to manage a colonic perforation surgically rather than endoscopically with endoscopic closure techniques is based on the type and location of injury, quality of the bowel preparation at the time of perforation, presence of an underlying colonic abnormality (eg, incomplete polyp resection, suspicion of malignancy within a polyp, or an obvious mass), clinical stability of the patient, available devices, and endoscopist expertise. Surgery is indicated in the presence of a perforation larger than 2 to 3 cm, the presence of diffuse peritonitis from gross feculent contamination, a concomitant bowel abnormality, and clinical deterioration despite optimal endoscopic and medical management.

When the bowel preparation is of high quality and the perforation is smaller than 1 to 2 cm, endoscopic management can be effective. However, it must be emphasized that prompt recognition and immediate endoscopic closure of the perforation itself are key determinants for a successful outcome.[9] The patient should be placed in a position so that the perforation is in a nondependent location, and suction of the affected and surrounding colonic segments should be performed to prevent fecal spillage into the peritoneal cavity. Carbon dioxide insufflation should be used instead of air, if available, and insufflation should be kept at a minimum to avoid creating or worsening a pneumoperitoneum and

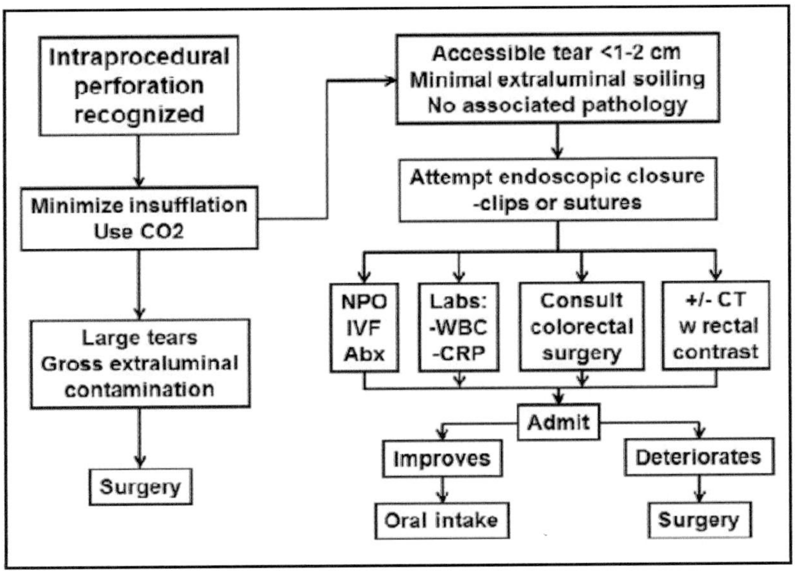

Figure 8-5. Suggested management algorithm for intraprocedurally recognized colonic perforation. Abbreviations: Abx, antibiotics; CRP, C-reactive protein; CT, computed tomography; IVF, intravenous fluids; NPO, nothing by mouth; WBC, white blood cells.

to lessen any potential egress of colonic contents through the perforation and into the intraperitoneal space.

Close clinical monitoring is essential after endoscopic closure. This includes serial abdominal examination to evaluate for peritonitis; frequent assessment of vital signs for tachycardia, tachypnea, and fever; and laboratory monitoring of inflammatory markers, including white blood cell (WBC) count and C-reactive protein (CRP) level (Figure 8-5). Ideally, the decision to proceed with surgery should be made within 24 hours after endoscopic closure if no significant clinical improvement is seen or in the presence of clinical deterioration because an additional time delay adversely affects surgical outcomes. This 24-hour window is based on studies of patients with colonoscopic perforations managed operatively; those who were seen later (more than 24 hours) were more likely to receive a colostomy rather than primary repair or single-stage resection with anastomosis.[4]

Endoscopic closure in the setting of a delayed perforation is controversial, and most experts consider late recognition of a perforation beyond 24 hours, with or without peritoneal signs, a contraindication to endoscopic therapy. Delayed endoscopic repair can be considered only if the patient's condition is stable and a specific site (eg, EMR) is highly suspected and easily within reach of the endoscope (eg, proximal rectum). Endoscopic management in this setting should be considered only in collaboration with surgical colleagues but may be warranted in select situations and in poor surgical candidates.

A difficult clinical situation is the delayed recognition of an undetected iatrogenic perforation at the time of colonoscopy. These are often discovered by subsequent radiologic imaging prompted by persistent or worsening pain in the postprocedural recovery unit. In many instances, such cases are a result of microperforations, and conservative management alone can be sufficient because such small perforations tend to close spontaneously by contraction of the colonic wall and sealing by pericolic tissue.[5] It is unknown whether prompt return to endoscopy for closure of radiologically proven microperforations results in better outcomes than either conservative or surgical management.

Table 8-1. Through-the-Scope Clip Devices

FEATURES	QUICKCLIP2 (OLYMPUS AMERICA, INC)	QUICKCLIPPRO (OLYMPUS AMERICA, INC)	RESOLUTION (BOSTON SCIENTIFIC CORPORATION)	INSTINCT (COOK MEDICAL)
Opened jaw span, mm	7 or 11	11	11	16
Rotation	Yes	Yes	Limited	Yes
Reopening capability	No	Yes	Yes	Yes
Median retention time, wk	2	Not available	4	Not available

Endoscopic Closure Devices and Techniques

Through-the-Scope Clips

Several 2-pronged, through-the-scope (TTS) clips are commercially available. These clips are manufactured by various vendors, and there are differences between these clips in terms of opened jaw span, rotational ability before deployment, and the capability to reopen the clip after closure but before final deployment (Table 8-1). To date, there are no comparative human studies that have established the superiority of one type of clip over another for closure of colonoscopic perforations or other indications. As a general rule, these clips are similar to each other in practice, and most experienced endoscopists can be equally adept at using any of these devices.

In general, TTS clips can be used to close perforations 2 cm or smaller despite the fact that successful closure of larger, nongaping perforations has been reported.[10] Successful closure depends on both the endoscopist and assistant. Familiarity with the use and handling of a particular TTS clip device is paramount.

The following maneuvers enhance successful clip application and closure:

- Application of gentle suction rather than forceful pushing of the clip into tissue to approximate the edges of the perforation and allow capture of a greater volume of tissue within the opened prongs of the clip
- Initiation of clip closure from left to right for a transverse perforation and from top to bottom for a longitudinal perforation
- Placement of closely stacked clips in a zipperlike fashion to ensure adequate closure (Figure 8-6)

Adjunctive techniques for closure of larger defects have been used, including the clip-endoloop and clip-omental patch methods.[11,12] The clip-endoloop method uses an endoloop to closely hold 2 or more clips in position. The clip-omental patch method refers to using clips to fasten a small omental patch over and around a perforation to aid healing. TTS clips can be especially effective in selected patients and have the potential to reduce

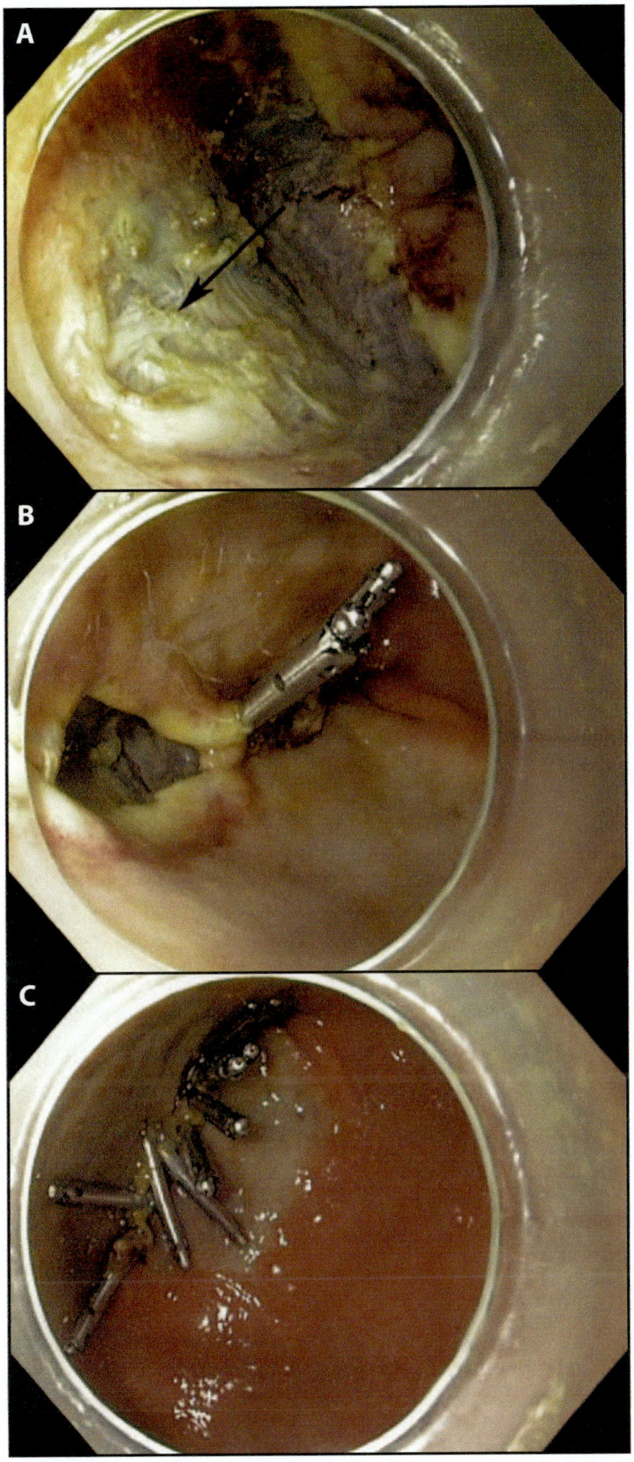

Figure 8-6. (A) Large ESD defect with injury to muscularis propria (B and C) closed using TTS clips in a zipperlike fashion.

cost and length of hospital stay compared with surgery.[13] Successful clinical outcomes after TTS clip closure of colonoscopic perforations vary from 59% to 93% in reported series.[10,14,15]

Although TTS clips can provide satisfactory closure of small perforations, they are often inadequate for closure of larger defects, particularly gaping holes rather than linear tears. This is because of their limited opening widths, low closing forces, and potential for early dislodgement. With the advent of Natural Orifice Translumenal Endoscopic Surgery (NOTES), techniques for enterotomy closure have been developed, including 2 devices recently approved by the US Food and Drug Administration (FDA): the Over-the-Scope Clip System (OTSC System; Ovesco Endoscopy AG) and the OverStitch Endoscopic Suturing System (Apollo Endosurgery).[16]

Over-the-Scope Clips

The design of the OTSC System is substantially different from that of TTS clips. This shape-memory nitinol clip has been compared with a bear trap. It is preloaded in an open state and mounted on a transparent cap that in turn is affixed to the tip of the endoscope. The setup and deployment of the OTSC System are analogous to those of traditional band ligation kits. With the application of suction, the outer edges of the perforation, with or without entrapment of adjacent serosal fat, are brought into the OTSC cap, and the clip is then deployed (Video 8-1). In addition to the use of suction, dedicated TTS grasping (twin grasper) or anchoring (tri-pronged) devices can be used to secure tissue margins and pull the defect into the cap before clip release. It is imperative that these grasping devices are fully retracted into the cap to prevent them from being captured inadvertently by the clip during deployment.

OTSC caps are available in different sizes (11, 12, and 14 mm) to fit endoscopes of various diameters, including adult diagnostic and therapeutic upper endoscopes and pediatric and adult colonoscopes. The OTSC clips are also available with 3 types of teeth, termed *atraumatic* (a), *traumatic* (t), and *gastrostomy closure* (gc). As a rule of thumb, the a-type clip with rounded teeth can be used for hemostasis, particularly in the thin-walled esophagus and colon, whereas the t-type clip with pointed teeth decreases the risk of clip slippage in indurated or fibrotic tissue and is used primarily for perforation and fistula closure. The gc-type clip, with long and sharp teeth, was designed for use in the thick-walled stomach. The OTSC System is FDA approved for closure of luminal perforations smaller than 20 mm.

The OTSC System enables more durable closure than TTS clips because of its ability to grasp more tissue and apply a greater compressive force for full-thickness closure. Perforated lesions with a high probability for successful OTSC closure are those smaller than 1 to 2 cm with healthy, noninflamed, nonischemic, and nonfibrotic tissue and for perforations treated within 24 hours of occurrence.[17] Poor closure response can be seen in patients with surrounding radiation-damaged tissue. In a prospective, multicenter study of 36 consecutive patients who had acute iatrogenic gastrointestinal tract perforations, sustained successful closure was achieved in 89% of patients.[18] In a recent systematic review of the OTSC System, the overall pooled estimates of technical and clinical success were 89% and 80%, respectively.[19]

Limitations of the OTSC System include the need to withdraw the endoscope to load the device (similar to a band ligator), the restricted field of view imposed by the cap, the potential for creating mucosal lacerations, the potential difficulty or impossibility of maneuvering the larger OTSC cap device through a narrowed and angulated lumen (as seen in the setting of left-sided diverticula), failure to access the perforation, and clip misfiring or misplacement during deployment. In the situation where a small perforation may be difficult to reidentify and where minimizing insufflation is important, placing a tattoo or TTS clip near the perforated site is recommended to facilitate its identification on reintroducing the OTSC-fitted endoscope. Caution must also be exercised to avoid inadvertent suction of extraluminal tissue or organ into the OTSC cap, except when an omental patch is desired.[20] Inadvertent complete luminal closure has been described when the OTSC was used in the small bowel. Although total occlusion of the colonic lumen by the OTSC is a theoretical possibility, this adverse event is less likely to occur given the larger luminal diameter of the colon.

The Padlock Clip (Aponos Medical) is another FDA-cleared over-the-scope clip device that showed reliable closure in a porcine survival study.[21]

Endoscopic Suturing

The OverStitch Endoscopic Suturing System requires mounting onto a specific double-channel endoscope (GIF 2T160; Olympus Corporation). The system consists of a curved needle with a detachable tip that carries a 2-0 polypropylene suture. The handle component of the device actuates needle transfer and movement of the suture arm, enabling passage and exit of the suture through tissue. The device is capable of deploying multiple running or interrupted sutures. A suture-cinching tool is used to tighten and secure the deployed suture.

As yet, there are no published clinical studies on the application of this device for closure of perforations in the colon, although there have been unpublished reports of its use to prophylactically close large rectal EMR and ESD defects deemed not amenable to clip closure for the purpose of preventing delayed perforation and bleeding (Figure 8-7). It is conceivable that perforations could be closed effectively with this suturing device, provided access to the lesion is straightforward (eg, rectal location). Device limitations include the need for a specialized double-channel endoscope, the inability to treat lesions beyond the reach of the dedicated endoscope, and restricted lesion access due to instrument design and colon anatomy. Additionally, the setup and learning curve are longer than with TTS and OTSC clips. This can be a deterrent when an acute perforation has occurred and when time is of the essence.

Other suturing devices may be forthcoming, as described in experimental settings and small case series. Unfortunately, these are not marketed currently for endoscopic closure.[16] Techniques that fashion inverted closure with serosa-to-serosa apposition (eg, staplers and the OTSC System) seem to provide superior closure compared with those that create everted closure with mucosa-to-mucosa apposition (eg, T-tags and pursestring suturing devices).[18]

Patient Monitoring After Endoscopic Closure

A multidisciplinary approach is essential in the postprocedural care of patients with a colonoscopic perforation. Initial management consists of bowel rest; intravenous fluids; broad-spectrum antibiotics; monitoring of vital signs and laboratory parameters, including serum WBC count and CRP level; and serial abdominal examination for the assessment of peritonitis.

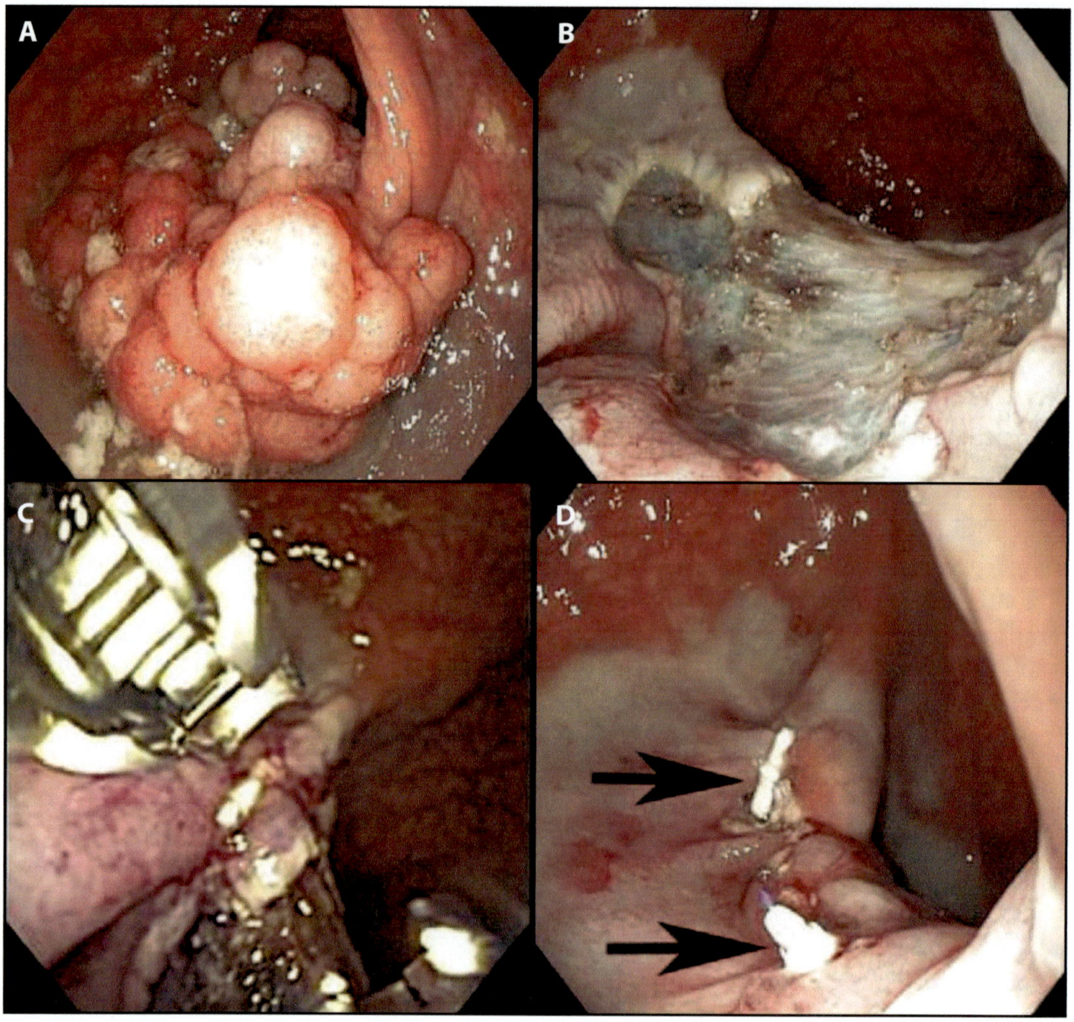

Figure 8-7. (A) Large rectal polyp (B) removed via ESD (C and D) with closure of the defect using endoscopic suturing.

Unfortunately, the endoscopic appearance of a secured closure is not predictive of long-term success because subsequent clip dislodgement or suture dehiscence can occur. This reinforces the need for close monitoring and early recognition of clinical deterioration. In some centers, a CT scan with rectally administered water-soluble contrast is routinely obtained to confirm the absence of leakage after endoscopic closure as part of an algorithmic approach to perforation closure.[22] However, there is a theoretic risk for increasing intraluminal colonic pressure with contrast instillation and opening the repaired site. If the patient clearly has not improved clinically, the decision to intervene surgically can be difficult, and surgery may be delayed beyond the optimal 24-hour period. Obtaining an abdominal CT scan in this situation can help guide decision making because the demonstration of extraluminal contrast or accumulation of fluid in the abdomen, or both, suggests ongoing leakage and should elicit prompt surgical exploration.

Oral intake can be resumed as soon as pain and fever subside, appetite and bowel function return, and laboratory markers of inflammation, such as an elevated WBC count and CRP level, improve. Patients whose course remains uneventful are typically able to resume a liquid diet 48 hours after the procedure with subsequent gradual advancement to solid food.

Conclusion

Surgery has been the mainstay in the management of colonoscopic perforations but may result in significant morbidity and mortality. With the advent of endoscopic closure techniques, endoscopists can use a more conservative approach in selected patients with perforations that are recognized immediately or early after a procedure, with minimal to no peritoneal contamination, and in the absence of concomitant colonic abnormalities that would require surgical resection. Prompt recognition and immediate closure of the perforation or site at high risk for perforation at the time of the procedure offer the best opportunity for a good outcome.

References

1. Panteris V, Haringsma J, Kuipers EJ. Colonoscopy perforation rate, mechanisms and outcome: from diagnostic to therapeutic colonoscopy. *Endoscopy.* 2009;41:941-951.
2. Lohsiriwat V. Colonoscopic perforation: incidence, risk factors, management and outcome. *World J Gastroenterol.* 2010;16:425-430.
3. Arora G, Mannalithara A, Singh G, et al. Risk of perforation from a colonoscopy in adults: a large population-based study. *Gastrointest Endosc.* 2009;69:654-664.
4. Iqbal CW, Cullinane DC, Schiller HJ, et al. Surgical management and outcomes of 165 colonoscopic perforations from a single institution. *Arch Surg.* 2008;143:701-707.
5. Yang DH, Byeon JS, Lee KH, et al. Is endoscopic closure with clips effective for both diagnostic and therapeutic colonoscopy-associated bowel perforation? *Surg Endosc.* 2010;24:1177-1185.
6. Avgerinos DV, Llaguna OH, Lo AY, Leitman IM. Evolving management of colonoscopic perforations. *J Gastrointest Surg.* 2008;12:1783-1789.
7. Baron TH, Wong Kee Song LM, Zielinski MD, et al. A comprehensive approach to the management of acute endoscopic perforations (with videos). *Gastrointest Endosc.* 2012;76:838-859.
8. Swan MP, Bourke MJ, Moss A, et al. The target sign: an endoscopic marker for the resection of the muscularis propria and potential perforation during colonic endoscopic mucosal resection. *Gastrointest Endosc.* 2010;73:79-85.
9. Raju GS, Saito Y, Matsuda T, et al. Endoscopic management of colonoscopic perforations (with videos). *Gastrointest Endosc.* 2011;74:1380-1388.
10. Trecca A, Gaj F, Gagliardi G. Our experience with endoscopic repair of large colonoscopic perforations and review of the literature. *Tech Coloproctol.* 2008;12:315-321.
11. Mocciaro F, Curcio G, Tarantino I, et al. Tulip bundle technique and fibrin glue injection: unusual treatment of colonic perforation. *World J Gastroenterol.* 2011;17:1088-1090.
12. Katsinelos P, Chatzimavroudis G, Zavos C, et al. Closure of an iatrogenic rectal perforation by using the Endoloop/clips technique. *Gastrointest Endosc.* 2009;70:405-406.
13. Magdeburg R, Collet P, Post S, Kaehler G. Endoclipping of iatrogenic colonic perforation to avoid surgery. *Surg Endosc.* 2008;22:1500-1504.
14. Cho SB, Lee WS, Joo YE, et al. Therapeutic options for iatrogenic colon perforation: feasibility of endoscopic clip closure and predictors of the need for early surgery. *Surg Endosc.* 2012;26:473-479.
15. Kim JS, Kim BW, Kim JI, et al. Endoscopic clip closure versus surgery for the treatment of iatrogenic colon perforations developed during diagnostic colonoscopy: a review of 115,285 patients. *Surg Endosc.* 2013;27:501-504.
16. Banerjee S, Barth BA, Bhat YM, et al. Endoscopic closure devices. *Gastrointest Endosc.* 2012;76:244-251.
17. Hagel AF, Naegel A, Lindner AS, et al. Over-the-scope clip application yields a high rate of closure in gastrointestinal perforations and may reduce emergency surgery. *J Gastrointest Surg.* 2012;16:2132–2138.

18. Voermans RP, Le Moine O, von Renteln D, et al. Efficacy of endoscopic closure of acute perforations of the gastrointestinal tract. *Clin Gastroenterol Hepatol.* 2012;10:603-608.
19. Weiland T, Fehlker M, Gottwald T, Schurr MO. Performance of the OTSC System in the endoscopic closure of iatrogenic gastrointestinal perforations: a systematic review. *Surg Endosc.* 2013;27(7):2258-2274.
20. Díez-Redondo P, Blanco JI, Lorenzo-Pelayo S, et al. A novel system for endoscopic closure of iatrogenic colon perforations using the Ovesco clip and omental patch. *Rev Esp Enferm Dig.* 2012;104:550-552.
21. Guarner-Argente C, Córdova H, Martínez-Pallí G, et al. Yes, we can: reliable colonic closure with the Padlock-G clip in a survival porcine study (with video). *Gastrointest Endosc.* 2010;72:841-844.
22. Kowalczyk L, Forsmark CE, Ben-David K, et al. Algorithm for the management of endoscopic perforations: a quality improvement project. *Am J Gastroenterol.* 2011;106:1022-1027.

Please visit www.routledge.com/9781617116148 to access additional material.

9

Colon Decompression

Robert E. Sedlack, MD, MHPE

It is not uncommon for a gastroenterologist to be asked to assist in the care of patients with large-bowel obstruction or pseudo-obstruction. Not all obstructions require endoscopic intervention. An understanding of the best management strategies for the many possible causes of obstruction will help guide one through the decision-making process and interventions offered. This chapter will review the common causes of this problem and the various decompression methods available.

Initial Evaluation

The most critical initial factors that dictate the timing and intervention to be used are the cause and duration of the obstructive symptoms. Acute mechanical obstructions, for example, may require expedient endoscopic or even surgical intervention to avoid catastrophic consequences, including perforation and peritonitis with resulting sepsis. However, patients with chronic motility disorders may have massive dilation of the colon lumen with little risk for acute perforation or even symptoms for that matter.

An accurate history is vital in all patients with known or suspected bowel obstruction. Patients with longstanding motility disorders are more likely seen to have a simple exacerbation of these underlying motility problems. More serious disorders, such as a volvulus, can still develop in these patients, and they should be evaluated carefully even if the underlying cause of their symptoms is suspected. In patients with an otherwise normal gastrointestinal history and among the elderly and those with a strong family history of colon cancer, the risk for acute obstruction resulting from a malignant neoplasm is significantly greater. Questions regarding recent changes in stool and gas output are

Adler DG, ed.
Core Concepts in Colonoscopy (pp 113-125).

also critical in helping one determine the degree of obstruction and the time course of the obstructive event itself.

Any initial evaluation should include fluid resuscitation, correction of any electrolyte imbalance, and strict bowel rest until the nature of the obstruction can be determined and resolved. A nasogastric tube can be placed if nausea, vomiting, or significant abdominal distention is observed. To reduce the resistance created by the rectal outlet, a rectal tube also can be placed to facilitate the passive evacuation of any gas or stool that moves to the rectum.

During physical examination, abdominal distention, tympany, and high-pitched or absent bowel sounds are the cardinal findings for both acute and chronic obstruction. As such, these findings are less helpful in determining the acuity of the situation. As a rule, the degree of discomfort patients experience during the physical examination can provide useful clues regarding their overall situation.

Among patients with abdominal distention, severe pain, fevers, rebound tenderness, or other peritoneal signs, endoscopic evaluation is generally contraindicated because of the risk of causing a perforation if it is not already present. In these patients, urgent surgical consultation combined with plain radiographic imaging to identify free abdominal air are critical maneuvers. The presence of a large abdominal hernia on examination should prompt one to consider the possibility that the patient has incarcerated or strangulated loops of small or large bowel, which also would warrant urgent surgical evaluation.

In less severe situations (eg, benign vital signs and the absence of peritoneal signs), further radiographic evaluation is often helpful. Plain radiographs are typically adequate for identifying acute volvulus or simply the degree of colonic luminal distention. If plain radiographs are indeterminate as to the degree, location, or cause of obstruction, computed tomography (CT) imaging can be helpful, as can water-soluble contrast enema studies. For patients who undergo enema studies, the high osmolarity of the water-soluble contrast also can be therapeutic in patients with an obstruction caused by fecal impaction because of its cathartic properties. In general, barium is not recommended for rectal contrast in patients with acute obstructions because of the possibility of compounding or prolonging the obstructive symptoms, especially in patients with fecal impaction. As a final resort, diagnostic endoscopic examination can aid in determining the cause and location of any obstruction. Endoscopy also can enable potential interventions, which will be discussed further in this chapter.

Benign Colonic Obstruction

Acute Colonic Pseudo-Obstruction

Acute colonic pseudo-obstruction (ACPO), or Ogilvie's syndrome, is one of the more common benign causes of large-bowel obstruction requiring decompression. The syndrome is characterized by the development of acute distention of the colon in the absence of any mechanical obstruction of the lumen. ACPO is believed to result from a sudden decrease in effective colonic peristalsis (colonic atonia) from the loss of autonomic regulation. This is seen predominantly in patients who have been admitted to the hospital and have severe medical illness (eg, sepsis, myocardial infarction, or respiratory failure)

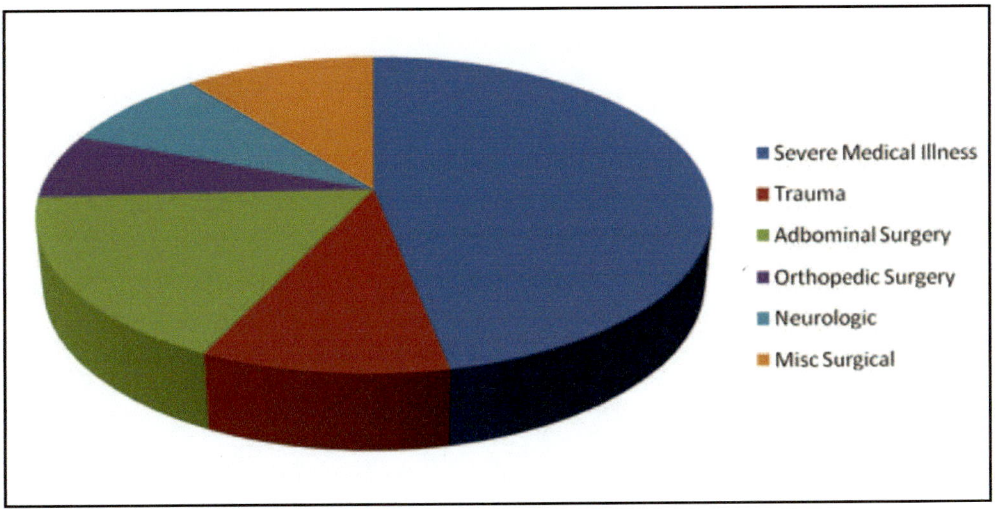

Figure 9-1. Underlying illnesses associated with ACPO.

and in the postsurgical setting, typically after abdominal surgery, orthopedic surgery, and cesarean delivery (Figure 9-1).[1]

ACPO can result in massive distention of the colon lumen. The high wall pressures can lead to ischemia of the colon wall and/or perforation (Figure 9-2). The presence of either complication increases the mortality of ACPO to as much as 40%.[2] Simple plain radiographs of the abdomen are frequently all that is necessary to confirm the diagnosis. ACPO is usually identified by significant distention of the colon lumen with the hallmark sign of gaseous distention down to the level of the rectum. If questions of a mechanical obstruction persist, a contrast enema should be considered. In the absence of an overt mechanical cause for obstruction and a cecum measuring 12 cm or more (or a transverse colon measuring 9 cm or more), therapy for decompression should be considered.

After initial supportive care, pharmacologic decompression with neostigmine is the first-line treatment for ACPO in patients without contraindications to such therapy. For those in whom pharmacologic attempts fail or who are not candidates for neostigmine, endoscopic decompression, with or without the placement of a deep colon decompression tube, should be considered. The specifics of these various methods are described in more detail later in this chapter.

Chronic colonic motility disorders rarely require acute decompression. Most respond to promotility agents and stool-softening regimens. However, severe cases can benefit from endoscopic intervention with placement of a percutaneous endoscopic cecostomy (PEC) tube for the purposes of venting.

Acute Volvulus

Volvulus of the colon results from the torsion of one of the freely mobile segments of the colon (typically sigmoid or cecum) and results in acute obstructive symptoms and potential bowel ischemia. Individuals at greatest risk for a colonic volvulus are those with longstanding institutionalization or paralysis (eg, paraplegia or quadriplegia), although a colonic volvulus can develop in otherwise normal patients as well.

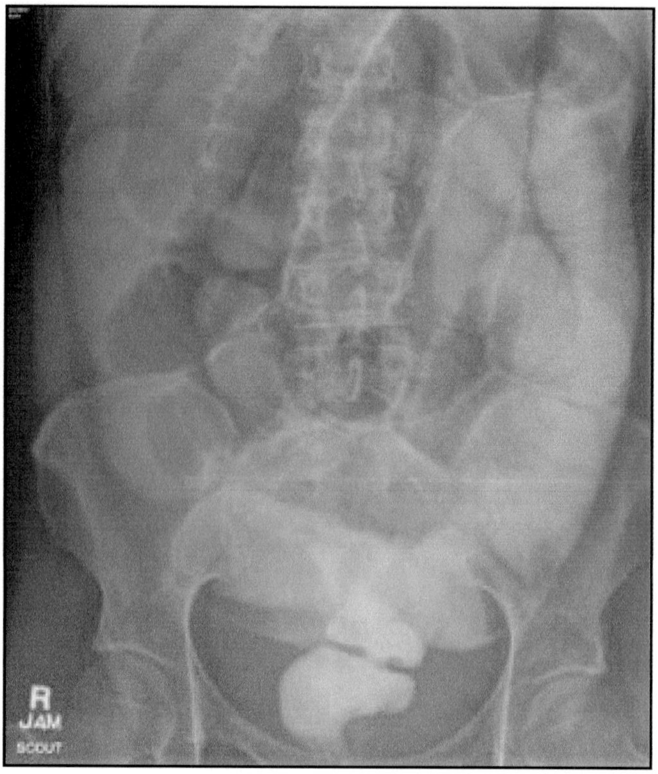

Figure 9-2. Plain abdominal radiograph shows significant dilation throughout the colon and even some loops of small bowel in the postoperative setting in a patient with chronic narcotic use.

Plain radiographs are often of great benefit in patients with a suspected colonic volvulus. The functionally closed section of the colon (cecum or sigmoid) will often manifest as a football-shaped area of lucency resulting from trapped air. As a general rule of thumb, the football will point to the area of concern (eg, a cecal volvulus will manifest on a plain radiographic image as a football whose inferior apex points to the right lower quadrant, whereas a sigmoid volvulus will be seen as a football whose inferior apex points to the left lower quadrant). This distended loop of large bowel also has been described as having a coffee bean shape, but the concept is the same (Figure 9-3).

Abdominal CT scanning is also helpful in the evaluation of suspected colonic volvulus. A CT scan can reveal the location of the volvulus, allow precise measurements of colonic distension, and detect torsion of vessels and mesentery around the bowel itself.

In an acute volvulus, endoscopic intervention can be beneficial in several ways. Colonoscopy can identify the exact location of the volvulus, evaluate the bowel wall for ischemia, and potentially reduce the volvulus itself. Endoscopically, a volvulus will generally appear as a twist or spiral in the colonic lumen; as a general rule, the endoscope can be advanced safely through this area (Figure 9-4). Often, just advancing the endoscope through the volvulus is sufficient to reduce it. If endoscopic reduction is achieved, the patient still needs close observation because recurrence of the volvulus is common. In many instances, placement of a decompression tube during endoscopy will prevent volvulus recurrence while the patient awaits definitive surgical intervention.

In patients with recurrent sigmoid volvulus who are not operative candidates because of comorbidities, placement of a PEC tube can be considered. The PEC tube will provide a location for the proximal colon to vent. In cases of cecal volvulus, a temporary tube (at

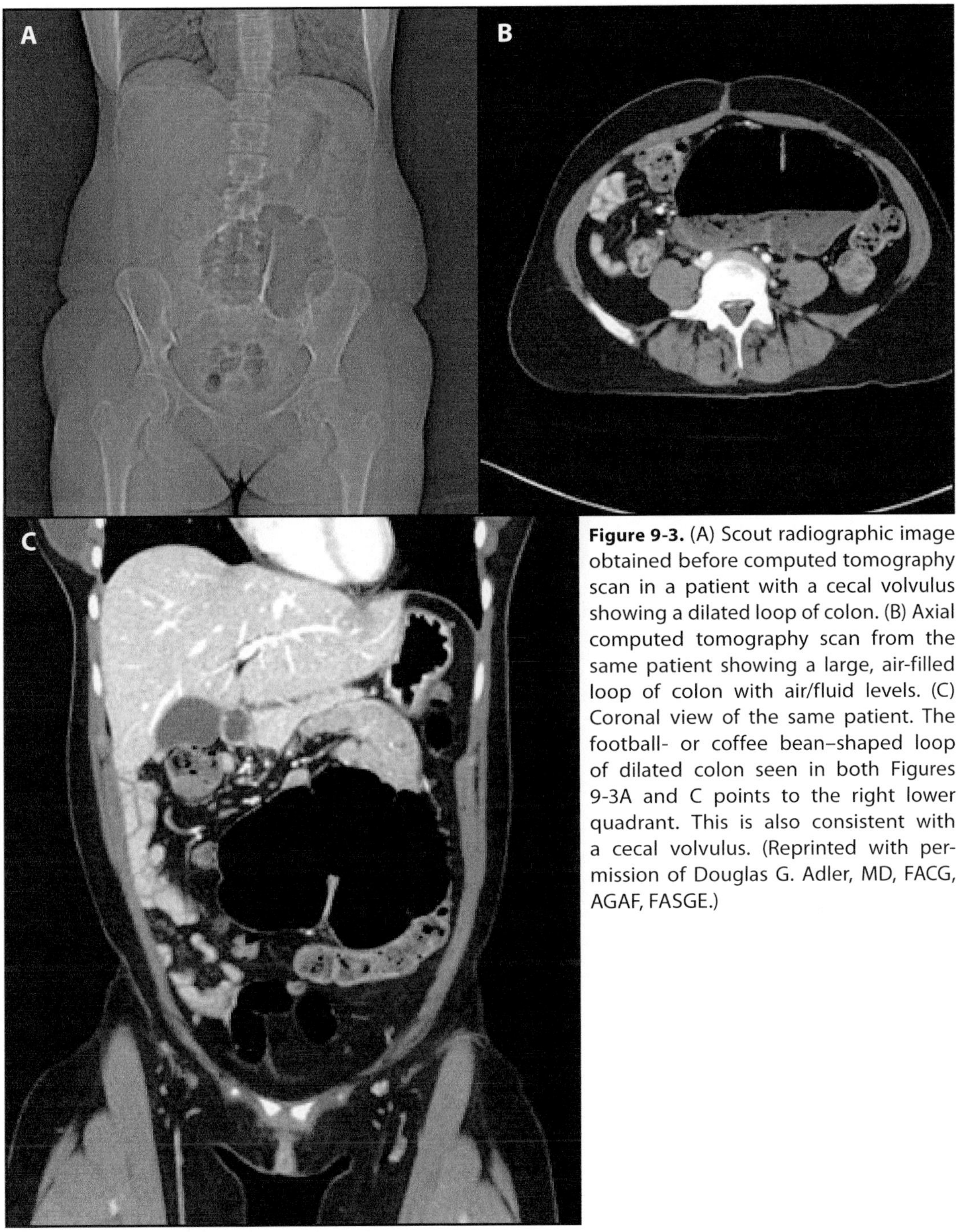

Figure 9-3. (A) Scout radiographic image obtained before computed tomography scan in a patient with a cecal volvulus showing a dilated loop of colon. (B) Axial computed tomography scan from the same patient showing a large, air-filled loop of colon with air/fluid levels. (C) Coronal view of the same patient. The football- or coffee bean–shaped loop of dilated colon seen in both Figures 9-3A and C points to the right lower quadrant. This is also consistent with a cecal volvulus. (Reprinted with permission of Douglas G. Adler, MD, FACG, AGAF, FASGE.)

least 6 weeks) PEC not only provides a location for venting, but it should create a fixed area of attachment between the cecum and abdominal wall, thus minimizing the risk of any future cecal volvulus.

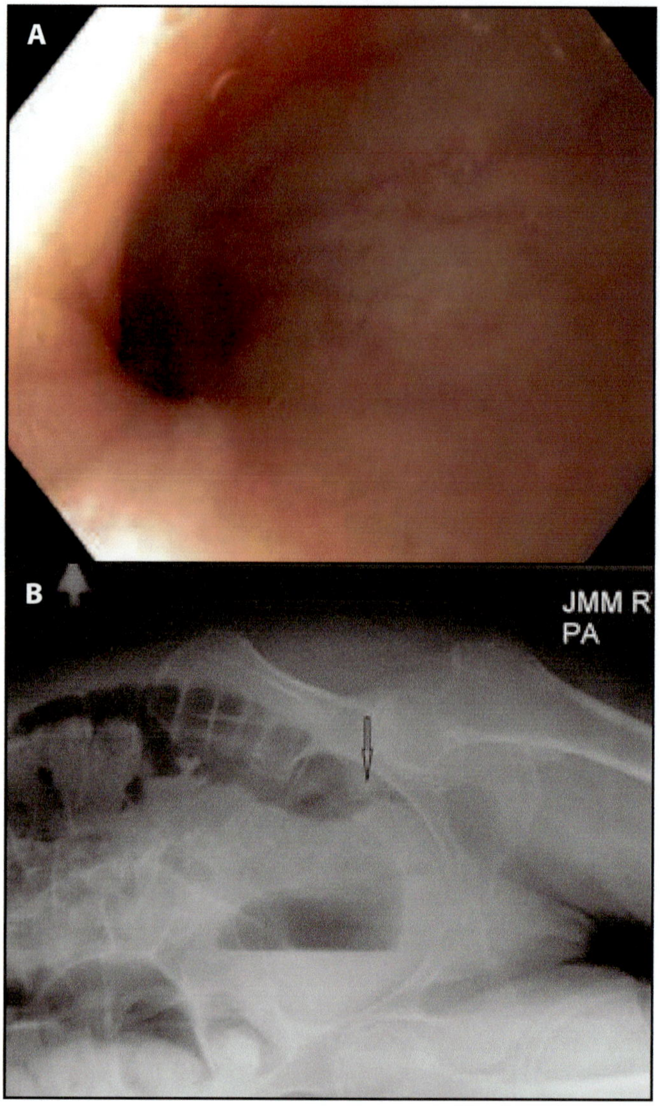

Figure 9-4. (A) The endoscopic view during colonoscopy shows a spiral turn consistent with a volvulus. (B) A radiographic image of a sigmoid volvulus showing a tapering of the dilated colonic gas pattern down to a bird's-beak appearance with no gas evident in the rectum. This finding could also be seen in a malignant obstruction.

Benign Stricture

Benign strictures in the colon can arise as a result of a number of disease processes, and some of these can lead to obstruction. Benign colonic strictures are caused most commonly by Crohn's disease, surgical anastomoses, or diverticulitis. Typically, acute decompression is not necessary for patients with benign strictures. These strictures tend to cause partial obstructions and gradually decompress themselves with conservative management, including bowel rest, nasogastric suctioning as necessary, and treatment of the underlying disease process with steroids or antibiotics if indicated. Once these measures have been applied, endoscopic intervention can be accomplished more safely, with better endoscopic visualization of the causative source and less risk of causing a perforation.

In cases of acute edema from Crohn's disease or acute diverticulitis, endoscopic management is frequently not required. For fibrotic strictures from these illnesses, endoscopic balloon dilation can help prevent recurrent obstruction. However, on occasion acute decompression may be necessary in patients with benign colonic strictures. In these instances, endoscopic therapy with balloon dilation with or without the placement of a colonic decompression tube will generally resolve the acute issue. If the stricture is refractory to conservative or endoscopic therapy, surgical intervention also must be considered. Pharmacologic therapy is generally contraindicated in all forms of mechanical obstruction.

Benign colonic strictures can be treated by endoscopic stenting in some situations. Stents tend to have the best effect in short-segment anastomotic strictures but can be used in diverticular strictures as well. Fully covered esophageal stents can be used in an off-label manner to provide durable dilation of the stricture itself. The stents can be removed at a later date with a rat-tooth forceps; in many cases the stents will spontaneously migrate out of the colon once the stricture resolves. Recurrence of the stricture can occur even after apparently successful stenting.

Incarcerated Hernia

Acute colonic obstruction due to the incarceration of a colon loop within a large ventral hernia is not common but requires immediate intervention. Diagnosis is typically based on physical examination combined with radiographic evidence of colonic dilation proximal to the herniation site. Endoscopic therapy is unlikely to be of much benefit, and any gas insufflated during attempted endoscopy may compound the problem and increase risks for perforation. Attempts at manual reduction of the hernia should be made immediately, although urgent surgical reduction and hernia repair are the primary means for treatment.

MALIGNANT COLONIC OBSTRUCTION

Most malignant colon obstructions arise from primary adenocarcinoma of the left colon, although proximal colonic obstructions occur as well.[3] Other common sources of malignant large-bowel obstruction are locally invasive metastases from adjacent organs, such as ovarian or bladder cancers. These lesions also typically affect the sigmoid or rectum either by direct invasion or extrinsic compression of the colon lumen.

Malignant obstruction has traditionally been managed by a surgical approach with diversion, resection, or both, as parts of a multistep-resection approach. However, in patients with acute malignant large-bowel obstruction, surgical intervention carries significant risks, with mortality rates as high as 10%.[4] As such, these acute obstructions are commonly managed with endoscopic intervention, typically with placement of a self-expanding metal stent (SEMS). SEMS placement provides a number of advantages compared with urgent surgery. In the case of resectable tumors, placement of a stent allows a 1-step surgical resection of the lesion rather than multistage surgery. SEMS placement with subsequent colonic decompression also provides time to safely stage the lesion before surgery. In those lesions eventually deemed unresectable, placement of SEMSs in the acute setting will palliate the lesion, potentially avoiding the need for surgical intervention.

In instances where stenting is not available or not believed to be technically feasible, endoscopic decompression can still be performed with the goal of placing a decompression tube over a wire into the colon proximal to the level of the obstruction. Balloon dilation of a colonic malignant tumor should generally be avoided because of the risk of perforation.

Procedures for Colon Decompression

Supportive Therapy

Supportive therapy should be initiated for all cases of obstruction. Frequently, supportive therapy is all that is required for patients who do not exhibit worrisome peritoneal signs, severe pain, or significant colonic distention (greater than 12 cm). These measures include bowel rest (nothing by mouth), nasogastric tube suctioning if nausea is present or colon distention is significant, intravenous hydration, and elimination of any medications that may be compounding the problem (eg, narcotics, anticholinergic medications, sedatives, or osmotic laxatives like lactulose). Ambulation or frequent position changes also are recommended. In some cases, rectal tube placement can also be of benefit by eliminating anal canal outlet resistance. In severe obstruction, enemas should generally be avoided because they can result in perforation in as many as 5% of patients.[2] However, in patients with large-bowel obstruction thought to result from fecal impaction, a radiographic enema with water-soluble contrast may not only help diagnose the cause of obstruction, but it can also be beneficial in relieving the problem itself.

Pharmacologic Decompression

After supportive care, pharmacologic decompression is the next line of therapy in those without contraindications. There are several pharmacologic options for the treatment of ACPO. The most common is the administration of intravenous neostigmine. In cases of ACPO that do not respond to a period of conservative therapy, neostigmine has been shown to be beneficial in controlled trials.[5] Neostigmine is a short-acting agent that promotes colonic peristalsis by both acetylcholinesterase inhibition and muscarinic receptor activation. The time to onset of effect is quite short; usually the patient passes gas within minutes of administration of neostigmine. In trials, 2 mg neostigmine administered intravenously during a period of 3 to 5 minutes had a 91% response rate within 4 to 5 minutes of administration.[5,6] Neostigmine application can be repeated for those who initially do not respond or those who do respond but have a relapse.[7]

Neostigmine infusion has a number of potentially significant side effects. These include symptomatic bradycardia, asystole, bronchospasm, and hypotension. Therefore, careful patient selection is critical. Patients with significant ischemic heart disease, underlying bradycardia or other dysrhythmia, active bronchospasm, or significant renal insufficiency are not candidates for neostigmine therapy. Infusion also is contraindicated during pregnancy, in patients with known or suspected ischemic bowel, or in patients with mechanical bowel obstructions (eg, malignant neoplasm or volvulus). Because of the potential side effects of neostigmine, any attempts at infusion should be performed in a monitored setting such as an intensive care unit with atropine at the bedside, as well as an external pacemaker/defibrillator immediately available in the event of a cardiac complication.

Because of the side-effect profile of neostigmine, newer pharmacologic options have been sought, resulting in the development of the new class of peripherally acting μ-opioid receptor antagonists, which include the medications methylnaltrexone and alvimopan. These medications have proved to be effective and are approved for treating or preventing narcotic-induced constipation and postoperative ileus.[8] Their use for the treatment of ACPO is not yet approved, but one case report has shown the subcutaneous administration of 12 mg of methylnaltrexone to be effective in an instance where opioids were involved and neostigmine treatment failed.[9] Because medications in this class do not act on central μ-receptors, narcotic pain control is not affected and withdrawal symptoms should not be precipitated in patients being treated with chronic narcotics. These medications also do not have the profound cardiovascular side effects seen with neostigmine. If additional research proves these options to be safe and effective for this indication, these may quickly become first-line pharmacologic therapy for colonic pseudo-obstruction where narcotics are involved.

The use of other traditional prokinetic agents (eg, metoclopramide or erythromycin) has been reported in patients with ACPO, but these are not used widely in this setting at this time.[10]

Simple Endoscopic Decompression

Endoscopic decompression is indicated for patients in whom supportive and/or pharmacologic therapy has failed or in whom pharmacologic therapy is contraindicated. Endoscopic decompression should not be attempted in patients with signs of peritonitis, perforation, or gangrenous bowel. Otherwise, for acute cases that have no fixed obstruction and where one-time decompression is all that is likely necessary, simple passage of a colonoscope into the proximal large bowel is performed. The goal is to reach the proximal transverse colon because cecal intubation is generally not required to decompress the right colon.

Because the colon is not prepared in these procedures and because of the already high wall tension in the colon, great care must be taken to minimize insufflation to avoid perforation. If available, carbon dioxide gas should be used instead of air for insufflation. Carbon dioxide will be reabsorbed gradually through the colonic wall, whereas standard air would remain trapped in the colon lumen. During scope withdrawal, simple suctioning of all trapped air is an effective means to reduce colon distention, improve the colonic blood flow, and reduce the risk of perforation from the obstruction. Successful decompression occurs in roughly 70% to 90% of patients.[11,12] Unfortunately, obstructions tend to recur in roughly 40% of patients after simple endoscopic decompression.[13] In such cases, or if suspicion is high that symptoms might recur, placing a decompression tube endoscopically would be indicated.

Decompression Tubes

Decompression tube placement is performed as an adjunct to simple endoscopic decompression (Figure 9-5). The addition of the tube is recommended for patients in whom the risk of recurrence is high (eg, narcotic use or volvulus) or if there are worries of colonic wall ischemia.[14] As with simple endoscopic decompression, the goal is to advance the scope only as far as needed to allow fluoroscopic advancement of a guidewire into the right colon. Once at the deepest point of insertion, the guidewire is advanced under fluoroscopic guidance into the ascending colon. The endoscope is then removed over the wire. As the scope is removed, attempts should be made to suction as much gas as possible from the colon. Once the endoscope has been removed, a sump-type decompression tube is then threaded over the guidewire and advanced under fluoroscopic guidance to the most proximal point possible. The wire is then removed from within the decompression tube (Video 9-1).

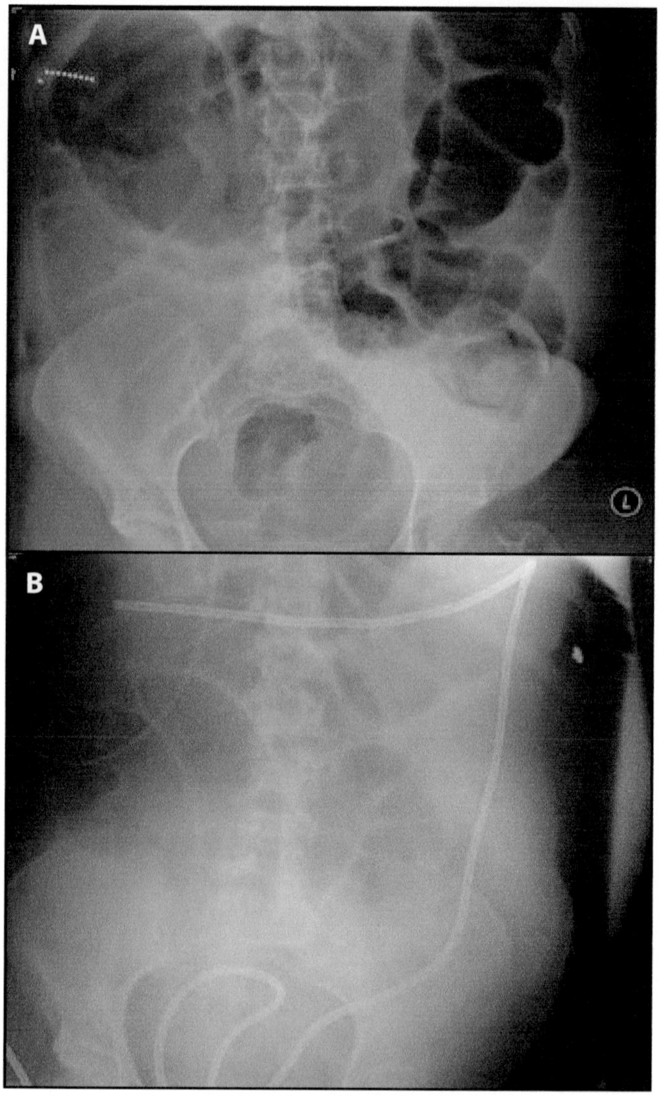

Figure 9-5. (A) Significantly distended colon in a patient with acute pseudo-obstruction before endoscopic decompression, along with (B) placement of a decompression tube with the tip near the hepatic flexure.

Decompression tubes come in several sizes, but the most common tube size is 14 Fr. A decompression tube kit is commercially available. The kit comes with the tube pre-loaded with an internal stiffening catheter. The tube itself and the stiffening catheter are advanced together as a single unit over the guidewire. Once in place, the wire and stiffening catheter are removed, and the decompression tube is connected to low intermittent suction. To maintain tube patency, this should be flushed with 20 to 30 mL water every 2 to 4 hours to prevent clogging.

In patients with malignant or mechanical obstructions, an endoscope may not always be able to traverse the obstructing process. Nonetheless, in most cases, a guidewire and decompression tube can still be advanced into the colon proximal to the obstruction. In nonmalignant obstructions, balloon dilation of the obstruction process also can be considered with or without tube placement, depending on the degree of success.

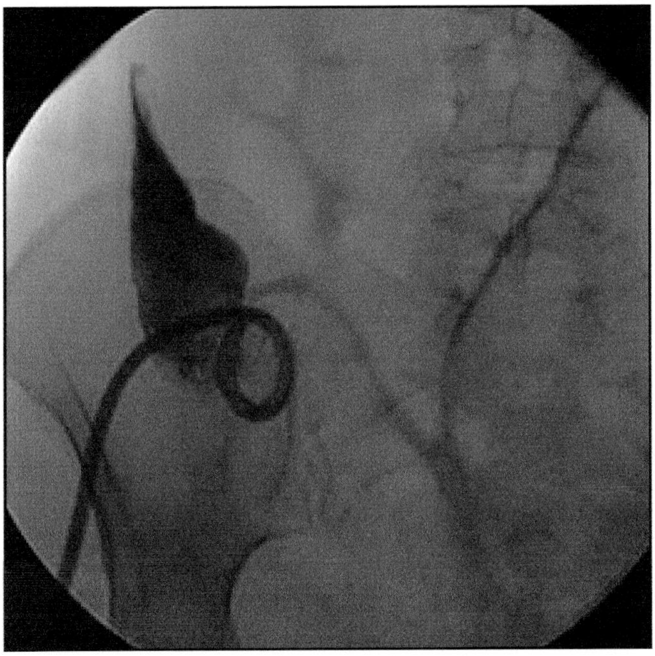

Figure 9-6. A pigtail cecostomy tube placed radiographically for colonic decompression.

Stent

Placement of SEMSs is commonly used in acute mechanical obstruction secondary to a malignant neoplasm. Details on stent selection and placement are covered in detail in Chapter 10. Generally, it is not advised to perform balloon dilation of malignant lesions because of the risk for colon perforation at the tumor site. Most stents continue to open gradually on their own during the 24 to 48 hours after placement.

Percutaneous Endoscopic Cecostomy Tube

For the purposes of chronic intermittent venting of the colon, a percutaneous cecostomy tube can be helpful.[15] This can be done by radiographic guidance with placement of a pigtail drain percutaneously into the cecum (Figure 9-6).[16] Endoscopic placement of PEC tubes is also possible.[17,18] Although not used frequently, this type of decompression tube uses a standard gastrostomy feeding tube kit and is placed during colonoscopy with or without the aid of fluoroscopy using a pull technique similar to that used for the placement of jejunal feeding tubes.

When placing a PEC tube, the endoscope is first passed through the colon to the cecum. The ideal location for tube placement is confirmed by both transillumination and external palpation with indentation. The site is marked, prepared, and draped in a sterile manner. Local anesthetic is used, and a seeker needle is advanced through the abdominal wall into the cecal lumen. This needle is grasped with a polypectomy snare internally to anchor the cecum against the abdominal wall while a catheter needle is advanced alongside the first needle through the abdominal wall into the cecum. The smaller needle is released from the snare, and the catheter needle, in turn, is grasped with the snare. With the introducer needle removed from the catheter, a loop wire is advanced through the catheter into the cecal lumen, and the wire is grasped with the snare and withdrawn through the colon and out the rectum. A standard feeding tube then is attached to the loop wire and pulled back up through the colon and cecum and through the abdominal wall, pulling the internal bumper up against the cecal and abdominal wall. The external bumper is fitted so that the internal bumper secures the cecal wall to the abdominal wall. The patient should receive preprocedure intravenous antibiotic coverage not only for typical skin flora, but also for fecal flora to reduce the risk of contamination of the wound.

Like other percutaneous feeding tubes, once placed, the PEC tube must remain in place for at least 6 weeks to allow the cecostomy tract to mature before tube removal or exchange are attempted. Because of the thin wall of the cecum, traction removal of original PEC tubes is generally not recommended. Instead, endoscopic removal is suggested to reduce the risk of cecostomy tract disruption. Once a balloon-type bumper replacement tube is in place, endoscopic intervention is no longer needed for removal or replacement.

Surgical Decompression

With any worrisome colonic obstruction, surgical consultation should be sought early because clinical deterioration can occur rapidly and progress to the point where surgical intervention is needed. Even if a surgeon is involved early, surgical intervention should always be considered a last resort in noncritical obstructions. Surgical intervention carries a greater risk than pharmacologic or endoscopic means of providing colonic decompression, with mortality rates as high as 6%.[2] However, in cases of severe obstruction accompanied by peritoneal signs, signs of necrotic bowel, fevers, clinical decompensation, peritoneal free air, or failure to respond to the measures outlined above, urgent surgical intervention is often indicated. Surgical decompression is typically accomplished by means of cecostomy, or, in cases of perforated or nonviable bowel, colectomy.

Conclusion

Early diagnosis is critical in the management of colonic obstruction regardless of the cause. Initiation of supportive therapy (ie, nothing by mouth, intravenous hydration, and possible nasogastric tube decompression) is indicated for all patients with an obstructive presentation.

Testing and management depend on the clinical picture and suspected cause. Frequently, supportive therapy alone is all that is necessary; however, medical or endoscopic therapy should not be delayed if symptoms do not improve. Additionally, surgical consultation should be sought early in the clinical course, and urgent surgical intervention should be performed at any time if bowel necrosis or perforation is suspected.

References

1. Geller A, Petersen BT, Gostout CJ. Endoscopic decompression for acute colonic pseudo-obstruction. *Gastrointest Endosc.* 1996;44:144-150.
2. Vanek VW, Al-Salti M. Acute pseudo-obstruction of the colon (Ogilvie's syndrome). An analysis of 400 cases. *Dis Colon Rectum.* 1986;29:203-212.
3. Repici A, Adler DG, Gibbs CM, Malesci A, Preatoni P, Baron TH. Stenting of the proximal colon in patients with malignant large bowel obstruction: techniques and outcomes. *Gastrointest Endosc.* 2007;66(5):940-944.

4. ASGE Standards of Practice Committee. The role of endoscopy in the management of patients with known and suspected colonic obstruction and pseudo-obstruction. *Gastrointest Endosc.* 2010;71:669-679.
5. Ponec RJ, Saunders MD, Kimmey MB. Neostigmine for the treatment of acute colonic pseudo-obstruction. *N Engl J Med.* 1999;341:137-141.
6. Saunders MD, Kimmey MB. Systematic review: acute colonic pseudo-obstruction. *Aliment Pharmacol Ther.* 2005;22:917-925.
7. Paran H, Silverberg D, Mayo A, et al. Treatment of acute pseudo-obstruction with neostigmine. *J Am Coll Surg.* 2000;190:315-318.
8. Becker G, Blum HE. Novel opioid antagonists for opioid-induced bowel dysfunction and postoperative ileus. *Lancet.* 2009;373:1198-1206.
9. Weinstock LB, Chang AC. Methylnaltrexone for treatment of acute colonic pseudo-obstruction. *J Clin Gastroenterol.* 2011;45:883-884.
10. MacColl C, MacCannell KL, Baylis B, et al. Treatment of acute colonic pseudo-obstruction (Ogilvie's syndrome) with cisapride. *Gastroenterology.* 1990;98:773-776.
11. Rex DK. Acute colonic pseudo-obstruction (Ogilvie's syndrome). *Gastroenterologist.* 1994;2:233-238.
12. Jetmore AB, Timmcke AE, Gathright JB, Hicks TC, Ray JE, Baker JW. Ogilvie's syndrome: colonoscopic decompression and analysis of predisposing factors. *Dis Colon Rectum.* 1992;35:1135-1142.
13. Saunders MD, Kimmey MB. Ogilvie's syndrome. In: McDonald JWD, Burroughs AK, Feagan BG, eds. *Evidence-Based Gastroenterology and Hepatology.* 2nd ed. Oxford, UK: Blackwell Publishing Ltd; 2007:303-310.
14. Geller A, Petersen BT, Gostout CJ. Endoscopic decompression for acute colonic pseudo-obstruction. *Gastrointest Endosc.* 1996;44:144-150.
15. Chevallier P, Marcy PY, Francois E, et al. Controlled transperitoneal percutaneous cecostomy as a therapeutic alternative to the endoscopic decompression for Ogilvie's syndrome. *Am J Gastroenterol.* 2002;97:471-474.
16. VanSonnenberg E, Varney RR, Casola G, et al. Percutaneous cecostomy for Ogilvie's syndrome: laboratory observations and clinical experience. *Radiology.* 1990;175:679-682.
17. Ramage JI, Baron TH. Percutaneous endoscopic cecostomy: a case series. *Gastrointest Endosc.* 2003;57:752-755.
18. Lynch CR, Jones RG, Hilden K, Wills JC, Fang JC. Percutaneous endoscopic cecostomy in adults: a case series. *Gastrointest Endosc.* 2006;64:279-282.

Please visit www.routledge.com/9781617116148 to access additional material.

10

Colonic Stenting
What You Need to Know

Kathryn R. Byrne, MD and Douglas G. Adler, MD, FACG, AGAF, FASGE

The self-expandable metal stent (SEMS) was placed endoscopically for the first time in 1992 for palliation of obstruction from rectal cancer.[1] Since that time, the use of expandable stents in the large bowel has broadened to multiple indications and use throughout the entire colon. Self-expanding stents are used most commonly to treat large-bowel obstructions, either from primary colorectal cancer or from extrinsic lesions, which are often metastatic in nature. Other possible uses of stents in the large bowel include treatment of anastomotic strictures and diverticular strictures. SEMSs can be used in the preoperative (as a bridge to surgery) and palliative settings in patients with primary colorectal cancers.

There are 2 main types of SEMS currently used: through-the-scope (TTS) stents and non–through-the-scope (non-TTS) stents. TTS stents are used most commonly. SEMSs that have been approved in the United States that are dedicated for colonic use are all uncovered because covered SEMSs have a high migration rate.

Technique: Step-by-Step Instructions on Stent Placement

Endoscopic stent placement in the colon can be technically difficult because of many factors. Tumors are often located at (or create) sharp angulations in the colon. Sometimes this can make complete endoscopic visualization of the tumor and lumen difficult.

The first step in colon stent placement is to review any available abdominal imaging and any prior colonoscopy reports. The endoscopist can choose an endoscope depending on the location of the lesion. In distal colonic tumors, a therapeutic upper endoscope or flexible sigmoidoscopy endoscope, both of which have a working channel that can

Adler DG, ed.
Core Concepts in Colonoscopy (pp 127-141).

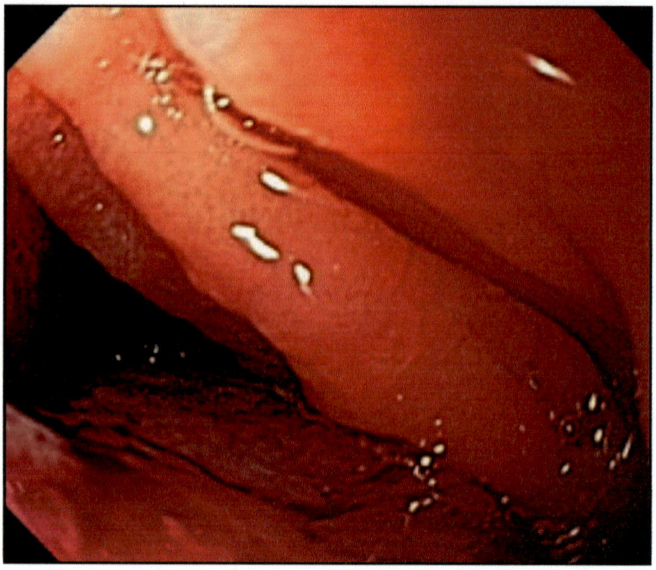

Figure 10-1. Endoscopic view of primary colon cancer causing intrinsic large-bowel obstruction.

accommodate a 10-Fr TTS endoscopic stent device, should be used. In proximal colonic tumors, an adult colonoscope will be required. A pediatric colonoscope or other thinner instrument can be used if the purpose of the endoscopy is only to place a guidewire for use by a non-TTS stent given its lack of a therapeutic working channel. In cases where the tumor creates or is located at a sharp angulation, a side-viewing endoscope (duodenoscope) can be used, although this is rarely necessary.

Once the endoscope is passed to the site of the tumor, the lesion can be inspected directly for any obvious residual lumen, signs of bleeding, ulceration, or other factors that may affect stent placement (Figure 10-1). Any signs of impending perforation (eg, ischemic bowel) should be noted because these may be indications to abort attempts at stenting. In general, there is no need to traverse the lesion. Advancement of the endoscope through the lesion typically offers little additional benefit, but this maneuver is not contraindicated if it can be performed in a minimally traumatic manner. In most instances, dilation of the stricture is not necessary before placement of a colon stent. Additionally, dilation of the stricture has been shown to increase the perforation risk.[2]

After the tumor site is visualized and inspected, a guidewire can then be passed through the working channel of the endoscope and then through the narrowed (or sometimes completely obstructed) lumen mass and into the proximal bowel. The guidewire itself is usually advanced through a straight biliary catheter (Figure 10-2). The guidewire is passed under both endoscopic and fluoroscopic guidance. The guidewires typically used to assist with colon stent placement have a floppy hydrophilic tip. Multiple guidewire sizes are available, although for colon stent placement, 0.025- or 0.035-inch-diameter wires are typically used. The increased stiffness of a 0.035-inch guidewire may provide greater stability as the stent is advanced across the stricture and may be beneficial for deployment of stents through sharply angulated strictures. However, 0.025-inch guidewires are more likely to traverse severe stenoses and may be advantageous for strictures with a complicated geometry and a tortuous lumen.

A retrospective study comparing the technical outcomes, clinical outcomes, and complication rates between 0.035- and 0.025-inch wires in 59 patients having 34 duodenal

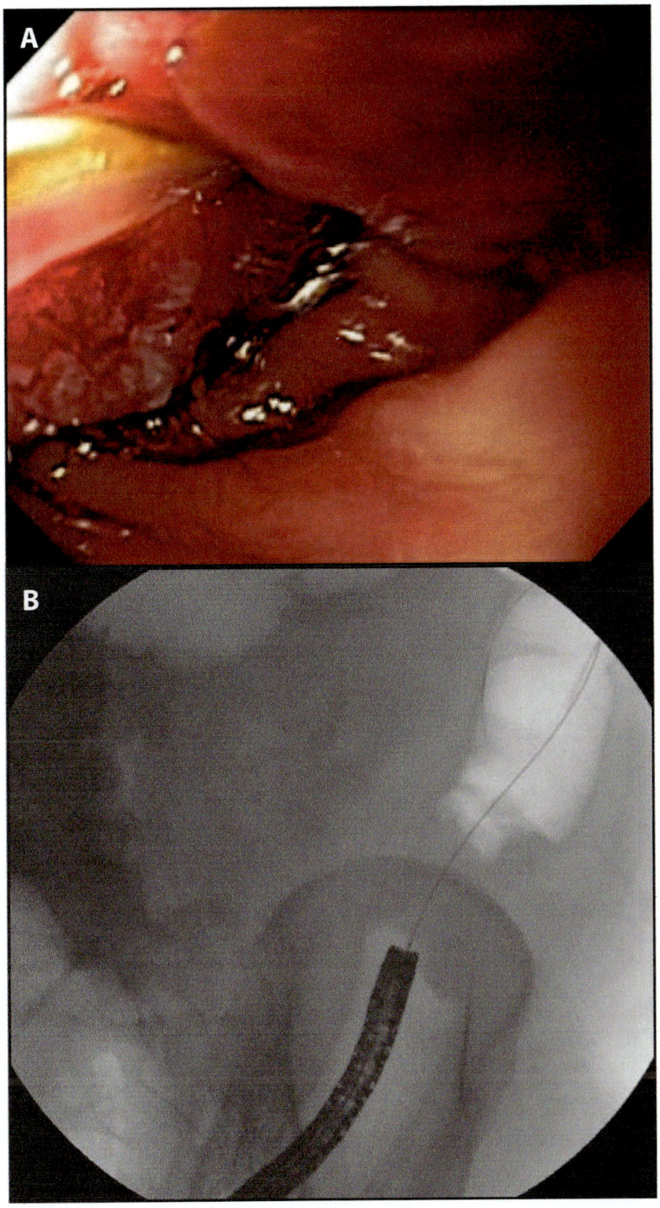

Figure 10-2. (A) A straight biliary catheter being used in the patient in Figure 10-1 to advance a biliary guidewire across the malignant stricture. (B) Fluoroscopic view of the guidewire advanced across the stricture and into the proximal large bowel. Image shows the air-filled sigmoid and descending colon.

and 30 colonic stent placements found that both wire sizes were equally safe and effective, arguing for operator selection at the time of the procedure, depending on personal preference and local tumor anatomy.[3]

The key to success in colon stent placement is being able to traverse the stricture with the guidewire, which can range from being straightforward to being technically difficult. Typically, a straight biliary catheter is placed through the working channel of the endoscope and then the guidewire is advanced through the biliary catheter and passed across the lesion. If the stricture is located at a sharp angulation and the wire cannot be passed, a clear cap (a soft plastic cap such as used in endoscopic mucosal resection/endoscopic mucosal dissection) can be used to obtain a more forward, direct view of the stricture. A

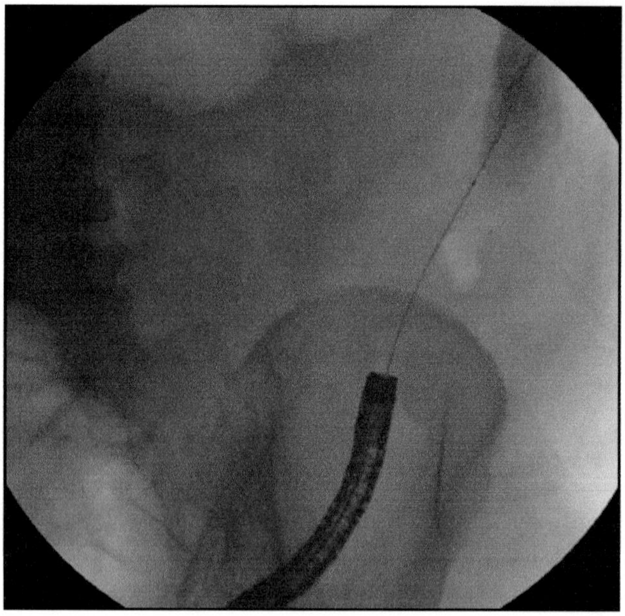

Figure 10-3. Fluoroscopic view of contrast injection showing dye in the proximal colon and a 3-cm-long large-bowel stricture.

sphincterotome also can be used to orient the catheter in the direction of the lumen if the lumen is angulated with respect to the stricture.[4]

Once the wire has traversed the stricture, the catheter can then be advanced over the wire and across the stricture and used to inject contrast to further define the length and geometry of the stricture (Figure 10-3). Using this information, the clinician should choose a stent long enough to bridge the entire stricture and extend at least 1 to 2 cm beyond each end of the lesion after stent deployment.

Stents are available in a variety of lengths and have different features, including distinctive radio-opaque markers, construction materials, delivery catheters, and deployment systems (Table 10-1). In choosing a stent of appropriate length, it is important to remember that the stent will shorten when it transitions from its predeployment to postdeployment state. The labeled stent size refers to the diameter and length at full stent expansion.

Most colon stents are placed with a TTS delivery system, although some stents are available in a non-TTS delivery system. Both TTS and non-TTS stents require placement of a guidewire across the stricture for proper use. For TTS stents, the guidewire is usually advanced across the stricture under combined endoscopic and fluoroscopic guidance. For non-TTS stents, the wire may be placed with endoscopic and/or fluoroscopic guidance.

It is worth noting that non-TTS delivery systems are typically used in patients with obstructions of the left colon or the rectum, whereas TTS stents can be placed anywhere in the colon. When a TTS SEMS is used, the predeployed stent and its delivery system are advanced over the wire, through the working channel of the endoscope, and across the stricture, and then deployed under endoscopic and fluoroscopic guidance. Non-TTS stents can be deployed under fluoroscopic guidance alone (much like many esophageal stents) or under combined endoscopic and fluoroscopic guidance if an endoscope is advanced next to the stent at the time of deployment.

The mechanism of removing the constraining device to deploy the stent varies slightly, depending on the manufacturer, but the principles are similar across devices and manufacturers. As the restraining sheath is withdrawn or allowed to unravel, the stent will

Table 10-1. Commercially Available Colonic Stents

MANU-FACTURER	STENT	DEPLOYED DIAMETER OF STENT BODY, MM	DEPLOYED LENGTH, MM	COVERING	DELIVERY SYSTEM
Boston Scientific	Ultraflex Precision Colonic Stent	5.7, 8.7, 11.7	25	Uncovered	Non-TTS
	Wallstent Colonic and Duodenal Endopros-thesis	20, 22	6, 9, 12	Uncovered	TTS
	WallFlex Colonic	22, 25	6, 9, 12	Uncovered	TTS
ELLA-CS	SX-ELLA	20, 22, 25	8.2, 9, 11.3, 13.5	Uncovered and fully covered	Non-TTS
EndoChoice	Bonastent	22, 24, 26	6, 8, 10	Uncovered and partially covered	TTS
Leufen Medical GmbH	Ecostent	30	8, 10	Uncovered	Non-TTS
Micro-Tech Europe	Micro-Tech Colon and Rectum Stent	25, 30	8, 10, 12	Uncovered and partially covered	TTS, non-TTS
M.I.Tech	Choostent Colon/ Rectum	22, 24		Fully covered	Non-TTS
	Hanarostent Colon/ Rectum	20, 22, 24	6, 7, 8, 9, 10, 11, 12, 13, 14, 15, 16	Uncovered and fully covered	TTS
S&G Biotech	EGIS Colorectal	20, 22	6, 8, 10, 12	Uncovered and covered	TTS
	Hercules SP Colorectal Stent Dual Type	28 outer, 18 inner	11, 13, 15, 17, 19 (outer)	Inner uncovered, outer partially covered	Non-TTS
Stentech Inc.	Silky Colorectal Stent	24, 26, 32	5, 6, 7, 8, 9, 10, 12, 14	Covered	Non-TTS

(continued)

Table 10-1 (Continued). Commercially Available Colonic Stents

MANU-FACTURER	STENT	DEPLOYED DIAMETER OF STENT BODY, MM	DEPLOYED LENGTH, MM	COVERING	DELIVERY SYSTEM
Taewoong Medical	ComVi Niti-S Enteral Colonic	18, 20	6, 8, 10, 12	Partially covered	TTS
	Niti-S Enteral Colonic (D type)	18, 20, 22, 24	6, 8, 10, 12	Uncovered	TTS
	Niti-S Enteral Colonic (head type)	18, 20	6, 8, 10, 12	Partially covered	TTS
Wilson-Cook Medical	Evolution Colonic	25	6, 8, 10	Uncovered	TTS
	Colonic Z-Stent	25	4, 6, 8, 10, 12	Uncovered	Non-TTS

expand in a proximal to distal fashion. Some stents are reconstrainable up to a certain point (referred to as the *point of no return* and often demarcated by a fluoroscopic marker). Once this point of no return has been surpassed, the stent can no longer be reconstrained back onto the delivery catheter.

Colonic stents should be deployed in a careful manner, with active communication between the endoscopist, assistant, and person operating the fluoroscope. The speed of the deployment is often variable, with innumerable small adjustments made during the process to ensure proper stent positioning (Figure 10-4). Once the stent is fully deployed, the delivery catheter and guidewire are removed from the patient (Figure 10-5). The final position of the stent should be checked carefully before the procedure is concluded. If the position of the stent is believed acceptable, the procedure is complete. If the stent has misdeployed, it often can be removed in short order with a rat-tooth forceps. If the stricture is longer than had been expected, a second stent can be placed (generally in an overlapping, stent-within-stent manner) to bridge the obstruction completely.

Use of Stents in the Preoperative Setting

It is estimated that as many as 20% of patients with colon cancer have acute obstruction when they are first seen.[5] Patients with acute right-sided colonic obstruction are typically treated with a 1-stage surgical resection with a primary anastomosis if possible. Options for patients with an acute left-sided colonic obstruction include the following: (1) an endoscopic colonic SEMS, as either palliation or a bridge to surgery; (2) loop colostomy or loop

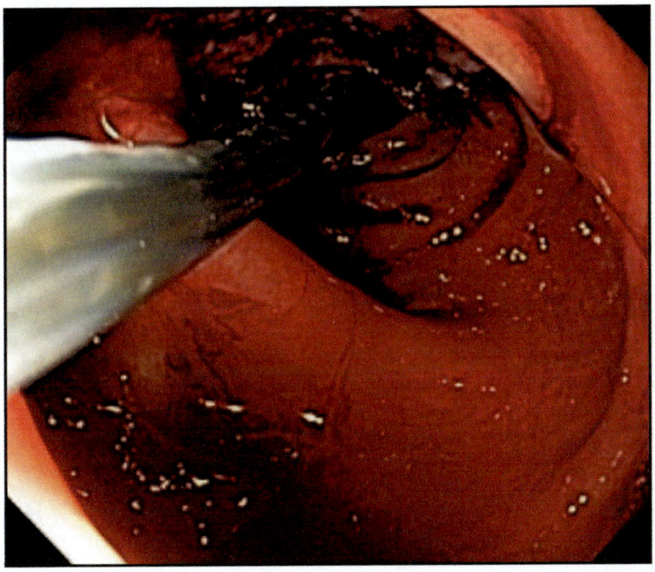

Figure 10-4. Endoscopic photograph illustrating stent deployment. The stent has been advanced over the guidewire, and the endoscope has been withdrawn slightly to allow better stent positioning.

ileostomy and subsequent resection (2- or 3-stage procedure); (3) primary resection with end colostomy/Hartmann's procedure; or (4) primary resection and anastomosis, with a total/subtotal colectomy or segmental colectomy with intraoperative colonic irrigation or manual decompression.[5]

In patients with acute left-sided colonic obstruction in whom a bowel preparation is not possible, placement of a colonic SEMS can be used as a bridge to a 1-stage surgery at a later time. Placement of a colonic SEMS as a bridge to surgery allows for a complete bowel preparation and then a single operation with a resection (the stent will be removed at the time of the surgery) and primary anastomosis, thus avoiding creation of an ostomy (Figure 10-6).

Other advantages of placement of a preoperative SEMS vs emergent surgery include a full preoperative medical evaluation and stabilization of any cardiac risk factors, and correction of volume status, electrolyte imbalance, and other issues before surgery. SEMS placement as a bridge to surgery may also allow time for complete oncologic staging by imaging and endoscopy to evaluate for possible synchronous lesions and other problems.

Numerous prospective studies demonstrate excellent technical and clinical success for preoperative SEMS placement for acute colonic obstruction.[5-11] Overall success rates are high, with technical success ranging from 75% to 100% and clinical success ranging from 84% to 100%.[2]

Many prospective studies have compared technical success rates, clinical success rates, complication rates, mortality, and length of hospital stay between patients with preoperative SEMS as a bridge to surgery vs surgery alone. A Cochrane meta-analysis reviewed 5 randomized trials including 207 total patients and compared outcomes between colonic stenting (102 patients) and emergent surgical decompression (105 patients) in patients with acute malignant colonic obstruction.[12] The technical success rate for SEMS placement among these 5 trials was 86%. The stent-related perforation rate was 5.88%, and the stent migration rate was 2.13%. There was no statistically significant difference in the overall complication rate or 30-day mortality rate between the 2 groups. Mean hospital stay was shorter in the colonic stent group (11.5 days) vs the emergency surgery group

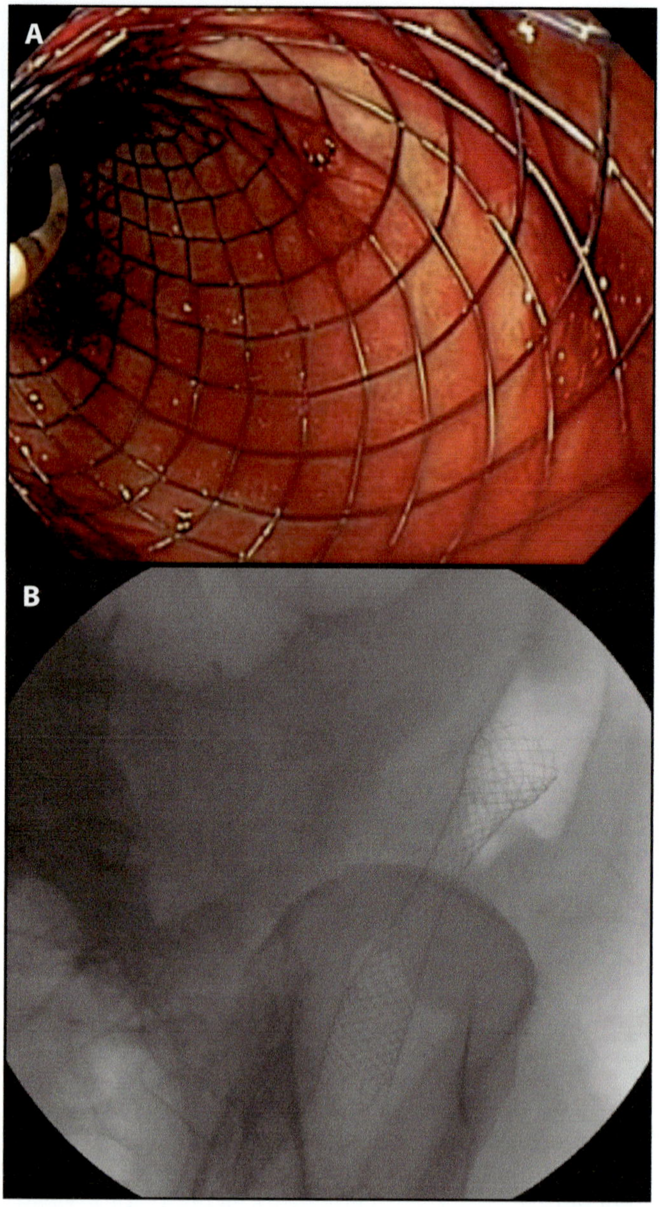

Figure 10-5. (A) Endoscopic image of the colon stent immediately after deployment. The inner portion of the stent-delivery system has not yet been removed. (B) Fluoroscopic image of the colonic stent after deployment and removal of the endoscope and all accessories.

(17.2 days). Another meta-analysis that reviewed 6 retrospective trials and 2 randomized trials compared outcomes between colon stent placement as a bridge to surgery vs emergency surgery in patients with obstructive colon cancer.[13] A decrease in overall mortality, postoperative anastamotic leaks, and initial stoma creation rates was reported in the group receiving SEMSs as a bridge to an elective surgery when compared with the group having emergent surgery. A meta-analysis performed at the Mayo Clinic evaluated 4 randomized trials comparing SEMS placement as a bridge to surgery (with vast variability in the rates of technical success of SEMS placement) vs emergent surgery.[14] In the studies with high technical success rates of SEMS placement, decreased overall complication rates were reported with SEMS placement as a bridge to surgery in comparison with emergent surgery.

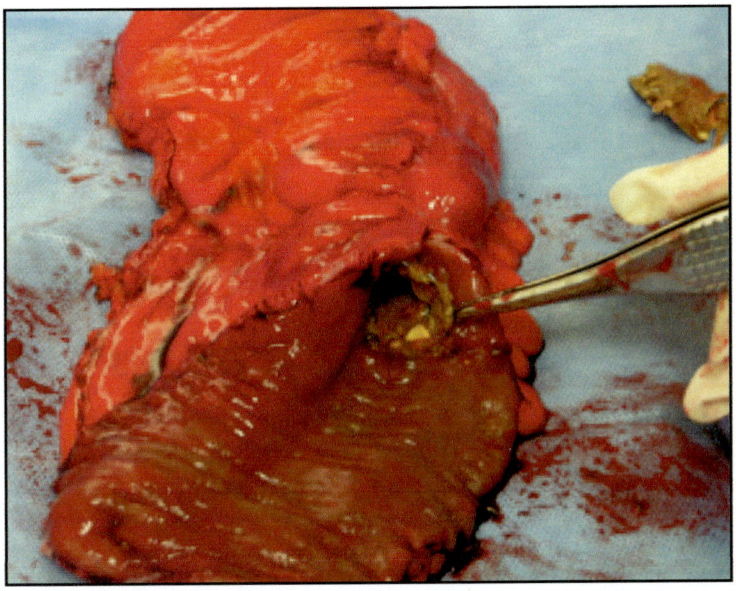

Figure 10-6. Surgical pathology image of a colonic stent and its surrounding colon cancer after en bloc resection.

Overall, the decision to place a colonic stent as a bridge to surgery vs emergent surgery in cases of acute colonic obstruction from cancer will depend on the expertise of the endoscopist and should be, if possible, a multidisciplinary decision based on coordination between the endoscopist, surgeon, and oncologist treating the patient.

Use of Stents in the Palliative Setting

Many patients with malignant large-bowel obstruction are not candidates for curative surgery secondary to metastatic disease or significant comorbid illnesses. SEMS placement in these patients as a palliative treatment can provide relief of obstruction and improve quality of life. As with the placement of SEMSs in the preoperative setting, there are high technical and clinical success rates in placement of SEMSs in the palliative setting.

It should be noted that colonic obstruction will develop in some patients with malignant tumors without a gastrointestinal origin (eg, bladder, ovarian, and uterine cancer) because of extrinsic compression by primary tumors or metastases. Often no tumor will be visible in these patients during colonoscopy, but they can have all of the same symptoms as patients with an obstructing colorectal cancer. Stents can be placed safely in these patients as well. In general, large-bowel strictures from extrinsic compression are often longer than those seen in patients with primary colorectal cancer (Figure 10-7).

A representative study of SEMS placement for palliation of malignant colonic obstruction in 44 patients showed a technical success rate of 95%, with a clinical success rate of 81%.[15] There were no perforations or SEMS-related deaths. Similarly, a study reviewing 168 palliative colon SEMS placements showed a technical success rate of 96%, 99% of which had immediate clinical success.[16] The median duration of stent patency was 145 days.

A large retrospective study involving 201 patients from 5 tertiary care centers evaluated outcomes of palliative SEMS placement for colorectal obstruction.[17] Technical success

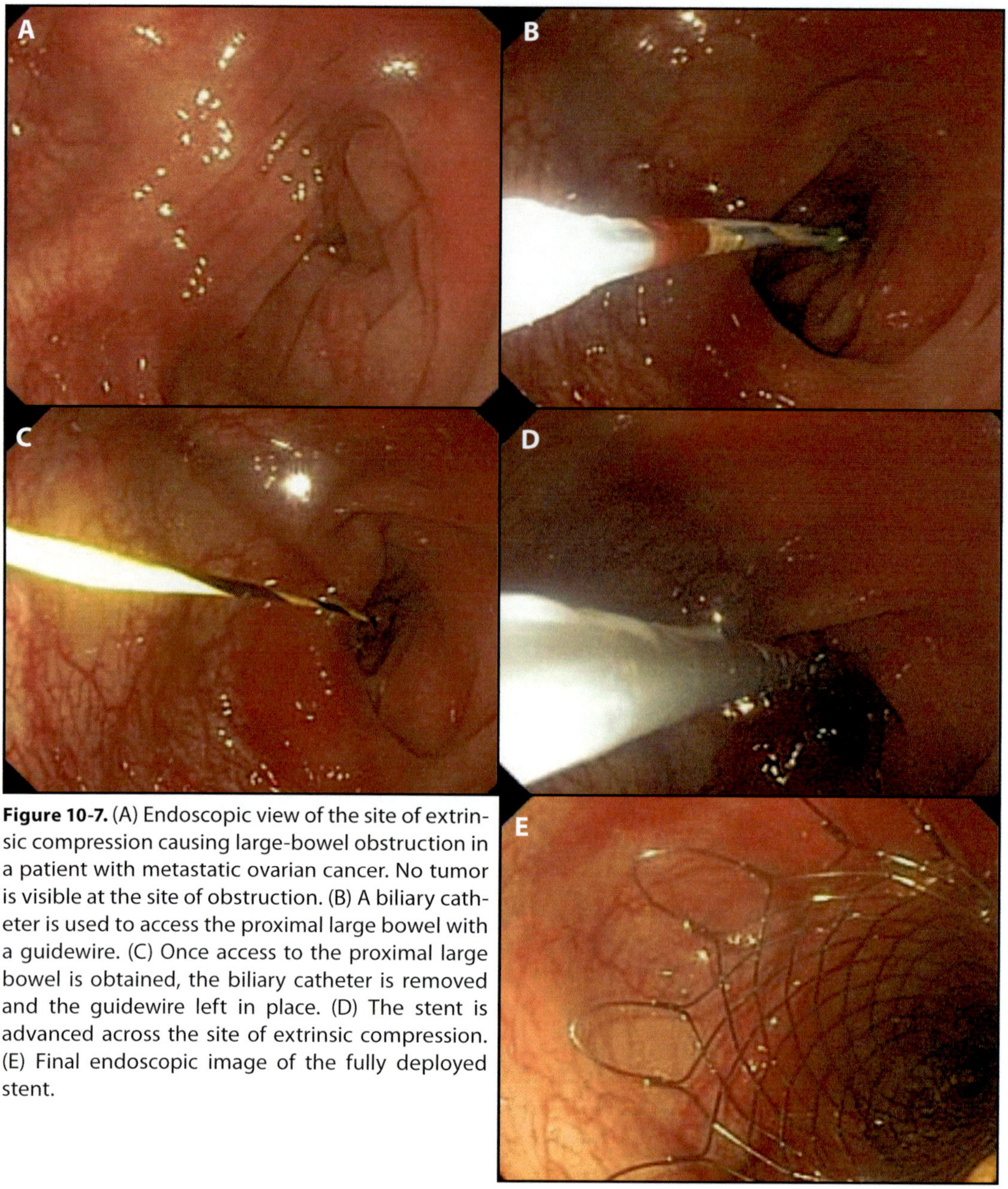

Figure 10-7. (A) Endoscopic view of the site of extrinsic compression causing large-bowel obstruction in a patient with metastatic ovarian cancer. No tumor is visible at the site of obstruction. (B) A biliary catheter is used to access the proximal large bowel with a guidewire. (C) Once access to the proximal large bowel is obtained, the biliary catheter is removed and the guidewire left in place. (D) The stent is advanced across the site of extrinsic compression. (E) Final endoscopic image of the fully deployed stent.

was achieved in 91.5% of patients and clinical success in 89.7% of patients. Seventy-five percent of patients were able to avoid colostomy placement. Major complications occurred in 11.9% of patients and included 11 migrations, 12 perforations, and 1 reobstruction. A key finding of this study was that the use of the humanized monoclonal antibody/angiogenesis inhibitor bevacizumab (Avastin) in these patients was thought to increase the risk of perforation by 19.6-fold. This is not an argument against the use of bevacizumab per se, but it is additional evidence that this agent can increase the risk of colonic perforation in patients with and without colonic stents.[18]

Although mature literature compares SEMS placement vs surgery in the preoperative setting, there are far fewer data comparing these options in the palliative setting. The one randomized trial of SEMS placement vs surgery in the palliative setting was discontinued prematurely secondary to a high number of perforations in the group receiving stents.[19] Ten patients were in the surgical treatment group and 11 patients in the group receiving SEMSs, with 6 perforations occurring in the group receiving SEMSs. The high perforation rate with SEMSs observed in this study has not been seen in other studies and is somewhat difficult to explain.

A different retrospective cohort study of 144 patients with unresectable metastatic colon cancer included 71 patients who had SEMS placement and 73 who had surgery. In this study, the group receiving SEMSs had lower rates of early complications (15.5% vs 32.9%, respectively).[20] Although the late-complication rate was higher in the group receiving SEMSs, the overall major complication rates were not significantly different. Of note, resection without anastomosis (stoma creation) was required in 39.7% of patients in the surgical group, a factor believed to potentially favor SEMS placement.

Another retrospective study reviewed 55 patients (29 SEMS placement, 26 surgery) who were treated in a palliative manner for left-sided colonic obstruction.[21] There were no immediate adverse events related to stent placement. Survival rates were similar between the 2 groups. The median hospital stay was significantly shorter in the group receiving SEMSs (4 days vs 13.5 days; $P < .0001$). Four patients in the group receiving SEMSs eventually required surgery (perforation in 2 patients, obstruction in 1 patient, and intractable tenesmus in 1 patient). Creation of a stoma was necessary in 12 of 26 patients in the surgical group and 4 of 29 patients in the group receiving SEMSs. This study showed that SEMSs provide effective treatment for palliative obstruction and are associated with less morbidity than palliative surgery, while having similar survival rates.

Stent placement in the palliative setting for malignant colonic obstruction is overall effective and safe. Patients having SEMS placement as an alternative to surgery for palliation are more likely to avoid creation of an ostomy. As with stent placement in the preoperative setting, the ultimate decision regarding SEMS placement vs surgery for palliation should be a multidisciplinary approach and will be influenced by the expertise at the institution.

Complications

Complications from colonic SEMS placement are generally divided into early (within 7 days) and late complications. Early complications include bleeding, perforation, stent misdeployment or deployment failure, and issues related to sedation. Delayed complications include stent occlusion from tumor ingrowth and/or overgrowth, perforation, stent migration, and bleeding. Stent migration may be partially attributed to the effects of chemotherapy, causing a reduction of the tumor size. Additionally, with placement of stents low in the rectum, there is the possibility of tenesmus and incontinence, although in practice, many patients can tolerate a low rectal stent, especially if the alternative is a permanent colostomy.

A large retrospective study analyzing long-term outcomes and complication rates among 168 patients having colonic SEMS placement for palliation of malignant obstruction demonstrated an overall complication rate of 24.4%, including both major and minor

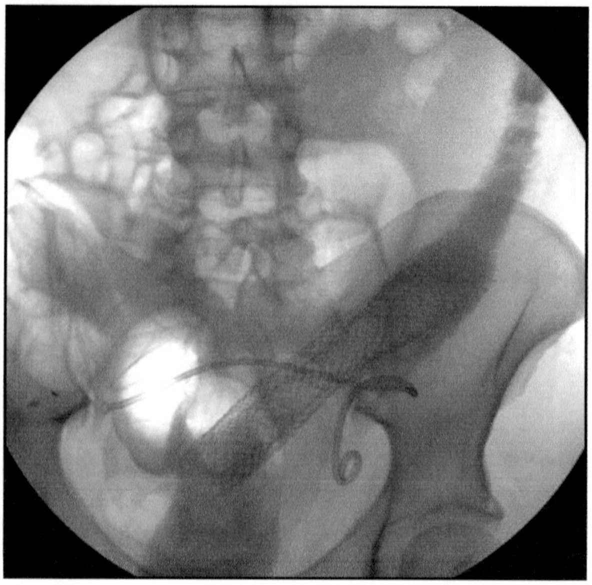

Figure 10-8. Fluoroscopic image of stent-within-stent deployment of a second colonic stent to treat tumor ingrowth through a previously placed colonic stent.

complications.[2] Complications included perforation (9% [3.6% procedure related, 5.4% stent induced]), occlusion (9%), migration (5%), and erosion/ulcer (2%). Sixty-five patients having colonic SEMS placement for malignant obstruction in the preoperative setting were evaluated, and 23.1% of patients had complications. Male sex, complete large-bowel obstruction, smaller stent diameter (22 mm or smaller), dilation of a stricture before SEMS insertion, and operator inexperience were all significant risk factors for complications. It is not entirely clear why a smaller stent diameter would potentially predispose a patient to complications, although this may be a surrogate marker for a more severe stenosis (ie, the endoscopist believed a larger stent would be too large). It also has been demonstrated by multiple studies that the use of bevacizumab therapy significantly increases the risk of delayed perforation.[19] This is not to say that patients should not receive bevacizumab for their malignant neoplasm, but that treatment with this agent may increase the overall risk from the stent.

Many complications resulting from SEMS placement can be managed endoscopically. Tumor ingrowth and/or overgrowth is usually managed with either tumor ablation via argon plasma coagulation, cryotherapy, or other methods or, most commonly, with the placement of a new stent inside the previously placed (obstructed) stent (Figure 10-8). In cases of stent migration, the original stent can be removed endoscopically, usually with a rat-tooth forceps, and a second stent then deployed across the obstruction if a new stent is believed to be clinically warranted. Surgery may be required in cases of failed endoscopic therapy and in patients who experience a perforation that cannot be closed endoscopically with clips or by other means.

Advanced Concepts and Techniques

There is far less literature on the placement of colonic stents for right-sided obstructive lesions than left-sided lesions. Historically, acute right-sided malignant obstructions were treated with immediate surgical resection and primary anastomosis. However, SEMS placement for proximal colon obstruction allows for elective surgery as opposed to emergent surgery and allows time for a preoperative medical evaluation and stabilization of any cardiac risk factors.

A multicenter study evaluating outcomes of SEMS placement in the proximal colon for treatment of malignant bowel obstruction in 21 patients showed that SEMSs appear to be both safe and effective.[22] Initial technical success was achieved in 95% of patients, with clinical success achieved in 85% of those patients. There were no procedure-related complications, and there was only one long-term complication from stent occlusion, caused by tumor ingrowth. Technical and clinical success rates in this study were comparable with rates seen with distal colonic stent placement.

SEMS placement in the distal rectum has the potential to cause tenesmus and incontinence, and SEMS placement within 5 cm of the anal verge has traditionally been regarded as a relative contraindication. A retrospective study investigated this issue by evaluating the technical success, clinical success, and safety of SEMS placement in patients with malignant rectal obstruction within 5 cm of the anal verge.[23] Records from 30 patients were reviewed, with 16 patients having obstruction within 5 cm of the anal verge (group A; range, 25 to 50 mm) and 14 patients having obstruction more than 5 cm from the anal verge (group B; range, 53 to 74 mm). The overall technical success rate was 100%. Ten (62.5%) patients in group A and 1 (7.1%) patient in group B reported pain. In 3 of the patients with pain in group A, the pain subsided spontaneously or was tolerated without the use of analgesics within 1 week after the procedure. The other 7 patients in group A and the 1 patient in group B who experienced pain required analgesics until death or elective surgery. The authors reported that the pain was tolerable in all 11 patients with or without the use of analgesics. Two patients in group A had fecal incontinence that had not been reported previously. There were 2 perforations in this study.

Overall, SEMS placement in the rectum is well tolerated by most patients and is an alternative to surgery and creation of an ostomy. Many patients will accept some degree of discomfort and the potential for some degree of fecal incontinence if it means avoiding an ostomy. If the SEMS is misdeployed too far distally, management options include immediate removal and reinsertion or the possibility of trimming the distal end of the stent with APC.

Although colonic stenting is typically performed to treat malignant obstruction, there are also potential uses in benign disease; however, published data regarding the use of colonic stents in patients with benign disease are limited. One case series successfully used Polyflex Esophageal Stents (Boston Scientific) to treat benign postoperative colonic strictures in 3 patients.[24] In 2 of the patients, the stent later migrated from the site of the stricture, and the patients remained without symptoms after that time. In the third patient, the stent was still in place after a 4-month follow-up period and the patient continued to have no symptoms. Another study retrospectively studied a total of 21 patients receiving SEMS placement for benign obstruction (8 with postsurgical anastomotic strictures, 2 with anastomotic strictures secondary to Crohn's disease, 10 with obstruction caused by diverticular disease, and 1 with a radiation-induced stricture).[25] Technical success was reported in 100% of patients and clinical success in 76% of patients. The overall complication rate was 43%, with most complications occurring in patients with diverticular strictures. The most common complication was perforation, which occurred in 6 patients. At the current time, it is fair to say that stent placement in the colon may be an option for patients with benign strictures, particularly in patients who are not surgical candidates.

Conclusion

Endoscopic stent placement in the colon can range from being straightforward to technically difficult because of many factors, including the degree of narrowing of the obstruction, the anatomy of the colon, and the angulation of the obstruction. Endoscopic SEMS placement is safe and effective overall, with high technical and clinical success rates.

SEMS placement as an alternative to surgery can relieve obstruction and improve quality of life, and it will be more likely to allow patients to avoid creation of an ostomy. Colonic SEMSs may be placed in patients with acute colonic obstruction as a bridge to a 1-stage surgery at a later time vs performing an emergent surgery, or the stent can simply be left in place as a palliative device if they have advanced disease or are not surgical candidates. The ultimate decision regarding endoscopic SEMS placement vs alternative therapies such as surgery should be a multidisciplinary approach and will be influenced by the expertise at each institution.

References

1. Spinelli P, Dal Fante M, Mancini A. Self-expanding mesh stent for endoscopic palliation of rectal obstructing tumors: a preliminary report. *Surg Endosc.* 1992;6(2):72-74.
2. Small AJ, Coelho-Prabhu N, Baron TH. Endoscopic placement of self-expandable metal stents for malignant colonic obstruction: long-term outcomes and complication factors. *Gastrointest Endosc.* 2010;71(3):560-572.
3. Chan J, Hilden K, Fang J, Adler DG. Duodenal and colonic stent placement with 0.025" and 0.035" guidewires is equally safe and effective. *Dig Dis Sci.* 2012;57(3):726-731.
4. Armstrong EM, Fox BM. Assistance of colorectal stent insertion by sphincterotome. *Dis Colon Rectum.* 2007;50(3):399-400.
5. Ansaloni L, Andersson RE, Bazzoli F, et al. Guidelines in the management of obstructing cancer of the left colon: consensus conference of the World Society of Emergency Surgery (WSES) and Peritoneum and Surgery (PnS) Society. *World J Emerg Surg.* 2010;5:29.
6. Brehant O, Fuks D, Bartoli E, Yzet T, Verhaeghe P, Regimbeau JM. Elective (planned) colectomy in patients with colorectal obstruction after placement of a self-expanding metallic stent as a bridge to surgery: the results of a prospective study. *Colorectal Dis.* 2009;11(2):178-183.
7. Cheung HY, Chung CC, Tsang WW, Wong JC, Yau KK, Li MK. Endolaparoscopic approach vs conventional open surgery in the treatment of obstructing left-sided colon cancer: a randomized controlled trial. *Arch Surg.* 2009;144(12):1127-1132.
8. Park IJ, Choi GS, Kang BM, et al. Comparison of one-stage managements of obstructing left-sided colon and rectal cancer: stent-laparoscopic approach vs. intraoperative colonic lavage. *J Gastrointest Surg.* 2009;13(5):960-965.
9. Jiménez-Pérez J, Casellas J, García-Cano J, et al. Colonic stenting as a bridge to surgery in malignant large-bowel obstruction: a report from two large multinational registries. *Am J Gastroenterol.* 2011;106(12):2174-2180.
10. Fregonese D, Naspetti R, Ferrer S, et al. Ultraflex precision colonic stent placement as a bridge to surgery in patients with malignant colon obstruction. *Gastrointest Endosc.* 2008;67(1):68-73.
11. Ng KC, Law WL, Lee YM, Choi HK, Seto CL, Ho JW. Self-expanding metallic stent as a bridge to surgery versus emergency resection for obstructing left-sided colorectal cancer: a case-matched study. *J Gastrointest Surg.* 2006;10(6):798-803.
12. Sagar J. Colorectal stents for the management of malignant colonic obstructions. *Cochrane Database Syst Rev.* 2011;(11):CD007378.
13. Zhang Y, Shi J, Shi B, Song CY, Xie WF, Chen YX. Self-expanding metallic stent as a bridge to surgery versus emergency surgery for obstructive colorectal cancer: a meta-analysis. *Surg Endosc.* 2012;26(1):110-119.

14. Dayyeh BK, Baron TH. Editorial: endoscopic stent placement as a bridge to surgery in malignant colorectal obstruction: a balance between study validity and real-world applicability. *Am J Gastroenterol.* 2011;106(12):2181-2182.
15. Repici A, Fregonese D, Costamagna G, et al. Ultraflex precision colonic stent placement for palliation of malignant colonic obstruction: a prospective multicenter study. *Gastrointest Endosc.* 2007;66(5):920-927.
16. Baron TH, Wong Kee Song LM, Repici A. Role of self-expandable stents for patients with colon cancer (with videos). *Gastrointest Endosc.* 2012;75(3):653-662.
17. Manes G, de Bellis M, Fuccio L, et al. Endoscopic palliation in patients with incurable malignant colorectal obstruction by means of self-expanding metal stent: analysis of results and predictors of outcomes in a large multicenter series. *Arch Surg.* 2011;146(10):1157-1162.
18. Sliesoraitis S, Tawfik B. Bevacizumab-induced bowel perforation. *J Am Osteopath Assoc.* 2011;111(7):437-441.
19. van Hooft JE, Fockens P, Marinelli AW, et al; Dutch Colorectal Stent Group. Early closure of a multicenter randomized clinical trial of endoscopic stenting versus surgery for stage IV left-sided colorectal cancer. *Endoscopy.* 2008;40(3):184-191.
20. Lee HJ, Hong SP, Cheon JH, et al. Long-term outcome of palliative therapy for malignant colorectal obstruction in patients with unresectable metastatic colorectal cancers: endoscopic stenting versus surgery. *Gastrointest Endosc.* 2011;73(3):535-542.
21. Faragher IG, Chaitowitz IM, Stupart DA. Long-term results of palliative stenting or surgery for incurable obstructing colon cancer. *Colorectal Dis.* 2008;10(7):668-672.
22. Repici A, Adler DG, Gibbs CM, Malesci A, Preatoni P, Baron TH. Stenting of the proximal colon in patients with malignant large bowel obstruction: techniques and outcomes. *Gastrointest Endosc.* 2007;66(5):940-944.
23. Song HY, Kim JH, Kim KR, et al. Malignant rectal obstruction within 5 cm of the anal verge: is there a role for expandable metallic stent placement? *Gastrointest Endosc.* 2008;68(4):713-720.
24. García-Cano J. Dilation of benign strictures in the esophagus and colon with the polyflex stent: a case series study. *Dig Dis Sci.* 2008;53(2):341-346.
25. Keränen I, Lepistö A, Udd M, Halttunen J, Kylänpää L. Outcome of patients after endoluminal stent placement for benign colorectal obstruction. *Scand J Gastroenterol.* 2010;45(6):725-731.

Please visit www.routledge.com/9781617116148 to access additional material.

11

Lower Gastrointestinal Bleeding
How to Evaluate and Manage

Linda S. Lee, MD and John R. Saltzman, MD, FACP, FACG, FASGE

Evaluation of Lower Gastrointestinal Bleeding

Clinical Evaluation

During the initial clinical evaluation of patients with any suspected gastrointestinal (GI) bleeding, including acute lower GI bleeding, resuscitation must proceed simultaneously with the placement of 2 large-bore peripheral catheters or a cordis catheter followed by administration of intravenous fluids (normal saline or lactated Ringer's solution), packed red blood cells (PRBCs), if indicated, or both.

Symptoms and Signs

When obtaining these patients' histories, one should focus on symptoms of hemodynamic compromise, including dyspnea, chest pain, lightheadedness, and fatigue, as well as potential causes of bleeding. The type and nature of the bleeding and key aspects of the history can also suggest a potential origin:

- Blood coating the stool suggests a distal source, such as hemorrhoidal bleeding, whereas blood mixed in the stool implies a more proximal source.
- Bloody diarrhea and tenesmus are associated with inflammatory bowel disease, especially if chronic, whereas acute onset of bloody diarrhea with fever and abdominal pain, especially with a recent travel history, suggests infectious colitis or ischemic colitis in a patient with a history of vascular disease.
- Pain with defecation occurs with hemorrhoids and anal fissure.

Adler DG, ed.
Core Concepts in Colonoscopy (pp 143-158).

- Change in stool caliber with associated weight loss is concerning for colon or rectal cancer.
- Abdominal pain can be associated with inflammatory bowel disease, infectious colitis, or ischemic colitis.
- Painless bleeding is characteristic of diverticular bleeding, arteriovenous malformation (AVM), and radiation proctitis.
- Nonsteroidal anti-inflammatory drug (NSAID) use is a risk factor for diverticular bleeding and NSAID-induced colonic ulcer.
- Recent colonoscopy with polypectomy suggests postpolypectomy bleeding.

Physical examination should focus on the following: orthostatic hypotension, which implies at least a 15% loss of blood volume; abdominal examination to palpate for tenderness, masses, peritoneal signs, liver span, and splenomegaly; and rectal examination, including inspecting the anus, palpating for masses, characterizing the stool color, and performing a stool guaiac card test.

Understanding definitions of the different types of bleeding is important when obtaining an accurate history and physical examination. Key terms to understand include the following:

- Hematochezia is defined as bright red blood from the rectum and usually implies a left-colonic source.
- Maroon stools are maroon-colored blood mixed with stool and often are associated with a right-colonic source of bleeding. Both hematochezia and maroon stools can result from a more brisk, proximal source of bleeding, including an upper GI source.
- Melena refers to black, tarry, foul-smelling stool that results from bacterial degradation of hemoglobin during a period of at least 14 hours. Although melena usually is associated with upper GI bleeding, it may occur with colonic bleeding if the source is very proximal. Ingestion of iron, bismuth, charcoal, and licorice should be excluded when considering a diagnosis of melena because these agents can turn stool black.
- Occult blood refers to the presence of small quantities of blood in the stool that can be detected only with a stool guaiac card test. Blood loss of at least 5 to 10 mL/day can be detected by stool guaiac card tests.

Laboratory Findings

Blood tests that should be performed include a complete blood count, international normalized ratio, electrolytes, and typing and cross-matching for blood products. Platelets should be maintained at levels greater than 50,000/mL, and coagulopathy should be corrected with vitamin K and/or fresh-frozen plasma. Vitamin K should be taken orally unless the patient has cirrhosis or biliary obstruction, in which case it should be administered subcutaneously. The full effect of vitamin K does not occur for 12 to 24 hours. Intravenous vitamin K reverses coagulopathy more quickly and may be used in cases of severe bleeding; however, patients should be monitored for anaphylaxis. Fresh-frozen plasma reverses coagulopathy immediately, with the effects lasting approximately 3 to 5 hours, and large volumes (greater than 2 to 3 L) may be required to completely reverse coagulopathy, depending on the initial prothrombin time. Recombinant activated factor VII (rFVIIa) has been approved for patients with hemophilia A and B with factor VIII

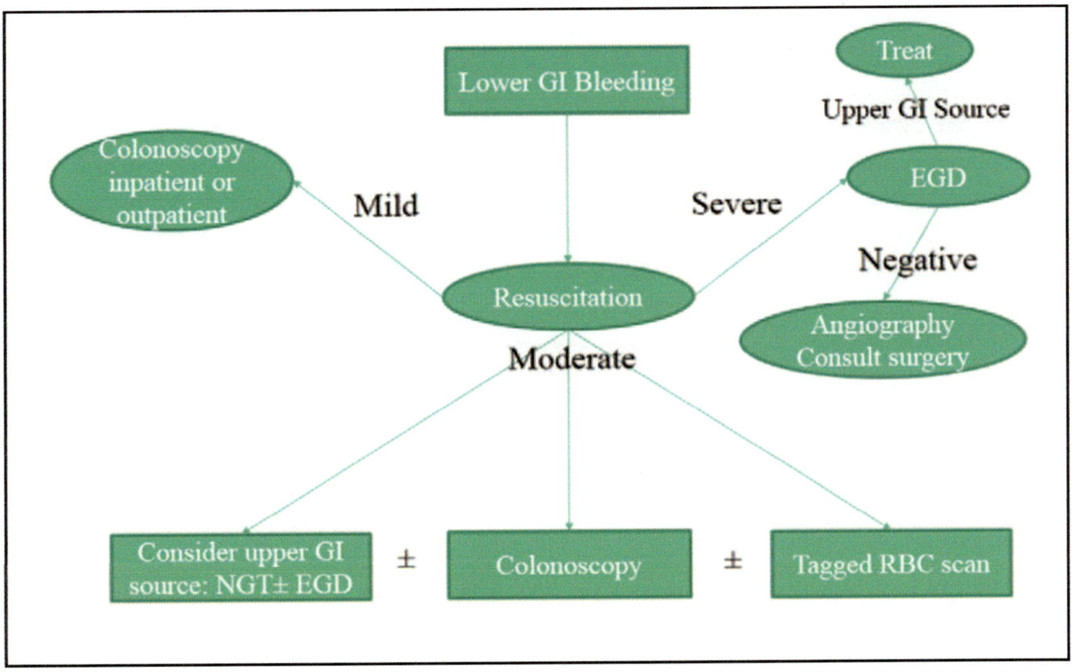

Figure 11-1. Algorithm for the management of patients with suspected lower GI bleeding. Abbreviations: EGD, esophagogastroduodenoscopy; NGT, nasogastric tube; RBC, red blood cell.

and IX inhibitors. Randomized trials using rFVIIa have not demonstrated a benefit to patients with cirrhosis with variceal bleeding.[1]

Diagnostic Approach

When patients are initially seen with lower GI bleeding, they should be triaged and treated based on the severity of the hemorrhage (Figure 11-1).

Patients with minor bleeding with scant hematochezia represent 75% to 90% of all patients with lower GI bleeding and may be evaluated as outpatients if they are clinically stable.[2] For patients older than 50 years, colonoscopy should be performed to evaluate for a potential source and screen for colorectal cancer. In younger patients, there is debate regarding the necessity of a colonoscopy vs flexible sigmoidoscopy. American Society for Gastrointestinal Endoscopy guidelines suggest that patients 40 years old or younger with scant hematochezia and without risk factors for colon cancer, anemia, or concerning symptoms such as weight loss should have flexible sigmoidoscopy, whereas older patients should be evaluated with a colonoscopy.

Patients may be seen with chronic intermittent bleeding that manifests as guaiac-positive stool, iron deficiency anemia, or both. These patients can usually be evaluated in the outpatient setting; however, if patients are severely anemic with cardiopulmonary symptoms or disease, inpatient admission should be considered for further monitoring, evaluation, and management. All of these patients should be evaluated with colonoscopy. If no source is identified on colonoscopy or if the patient has upper GI symptoms, an upper endoscopy should be performed. Abnormalities are seen during upper endoscopy in 25% to 41% of patients without symptoms.

Other patients with lower GI bleeding include those with episodic severe bleeding and continuous active bleeding who must be evaluated in the hospital. It is important to remember that approximately 10% to 15% of cases initially thought to represent lower GI bleeding are ultimately found to have an upper GI source. Clues to the presence of a possible upper GI source include hematochezia with hemodynamic instability, melena, and a history of upper GI bleeding. Placement of a nasogastric tube with possible nasogastric lavage or a prompt upper endoscopy should be performed to rule out an upper GI source in patients with severe lower GI bleeding.

Diagnostic Tests

Diagnostic evaluation must be performed only after patients have been resuscitated adequately. If an upper GI source is suspected, an upper endoscopy should be performed first. Lower GI evaluation can be performed with anoscopy, flexible sigmoidoscopy, colonoscopy, and various radiologic studies.

Anoscopy

Anoscopy is useful only for diagnosing bleeding sources from the anorectal junction and anal canal, including internal hemorrhoids and anal fissures. It is superior to flexible sigmoidoscopy for detecting hemorrhoids in an outpatient setting and can be performed quickly in the office or at the bedside as an adjunct to flexible sigmoidoscopy or colonoscopy. Unless a definitive bleeding source is found on anoscopy, additional testing is warranted.

Flexible Sigmoidoscopy

Flexible sigmoidoscopy visualizes the left colon and can be performed without sedation and with only minimal preparation with enemas. However, the diagnostic yield of flexible sigmoidoscopy in acute lower GI bleeding is only 9%. The role of anoscopy and flexible sigmoidoscopy among inpatients with acute lower GI bleeding is limited because most inpatients undergo colonoscopy.

Colonoscopy

Colonoscopy is the test of choice in most patients with lower GI bleeding because it is generally safe and may be both diagnostic and therapeutic. The diagnostic yield of colonoscopy in lower GI bleeding ranges from 74% to 100%.[3] Rates of detecting stigmata of hemorrhage (eg, active bleeding, nonbleeding visible vessel, or adherent clot) are lower at 22% to 42%.

The overall complication rate of colonoscopy in acute lower GI bleeding is 0.3% to 1.3%, with perforation being the most common significant event.[3] The complication rate of colonoscopy in an unprepared colon tends to be higher and the diagnostic yield lower. Bowel preparation is safe and well tolerated in most patients. In patients believed to be at risk of aspiration or fluid overload, the preparation should be administered cautiously. Between 4 and 8 L of a balanced electrolyte-polyethylene glycol (PEG) preparation should be delivered orally or by a nasogastric tube until the effluent is clear. Antiemetics and prokinetic agents such as metoclopramide 10 mg should be provided as needed during the preparation, especially if rapid delivery and a large volume of a PEG preparation solution are required.

Multiple validated scoring systems exist to predict the probability of rebleeding, surgery, and mortality in upper GI bleeding. This enables appropriate triage, aggressive management of high-risk patients, and potentially early discharge of low-risk patients. Few studies have stratified patients by severity of lower GI bleeding. The strongest risk factors identified for mortality in lower GI bleeding are advanced age, intestinal ischemia, and 2 or more comorbidities.[4,5]

It is not clear whether aggressive treatment with urgent colonoscopy improves outcome in patients with severe lower GI bleeding. Two small prospective trials of patients with significant lower GI bleeding randomly assigned patients to receive standard care or urgent colonoscopy.[6,7] Patients in the standard care arm had elective colonoscopy within 4 days of admission, whereas patients having urgent colonoscopy received 4 to 6 L of a PEG preparation solution orally or by a nasogastric tube during a period of 3 to 4 hours and had colonoscopy within 8 to 12 hours of admission to the hospital or diagnosis of hematochezia. More sources of bleeding were identified in the urgent colonoscopy arm in one study, but there was no difference in early or late rebleeding, length of hospital stay, surgery, mortality, or complications in either study. Therefore, the current data suggest urgent colonoscopy does not influence patient outcomes despite the increased identification of a source of bleeding, but larger studies on this topic are needed.

Tagged Red Blood Cell Scan

Tagged red blood cell (RBC) scans coupled with therapeutic angiography may be the test of choice in patients with massive lower GI bleeding that prevents colonoscopy, in those with ongoing bleeding and a colonoscopy with normal findings, or in those who have not yet been prepared for a colonoscopy and have suspected active bleeding. Although a tagged RBC scan is a purely diagnostic examination, angiography, like colonoscopy, can be both diagnostic and therapeutic.

A bleeding rate of at least 0.1 to 0.5 mL/min is required for detection by a tagged RBC scan. An injected radiotracer circulates in the blood, and extravasation of blood into the GI lumen can be identified on a series of images captured after injection (Figure 11-2). The most commonly used radiotracer for a tagged RBC scan—a technetium 99m–labeled RBC scan—involves labeling the patient's own RBCs in vitro and then reinjecting them into the patient. The RBCs persist for at least 24 hours in the circulation, which allows for longer and repeated imaging if the patient rebleeds during this time. Typically, a 90-minute imaging period is used because the diagnostic yield plateaus at this time. Approximately 45% of tagged RBC scans for lower GI bleeding have positive results. The bleeding site is localized accurately in 24% to 91% of cases—a broad range that may be due to different protocols and different types of patients. Scans with positive results within 2 hours have a higher accuracy in localizing the bleeding site compared with those showing positive results after 2 hours (95% to 100% vs 57% to 67%, respectively). With the relatively high rate of incorrect localization, confirmatory studies are required before proceeding to surgery.

Obtaining a tagged RBC scan before angiography enables the selection of patients who are bleeding sufficiently to have an angiogram and may allow more targeted use of angiography. A tagged RBC scan with positive results increases the diagnostic yield of angiography 2.4 times by excluding patients who are not actively bleeding. It is important to perform urgent angiography within 1 hour of a positive tagged RBC scan. Delaying angiography may increase negative results because lower GI bleeding is often episodic and intermittent.

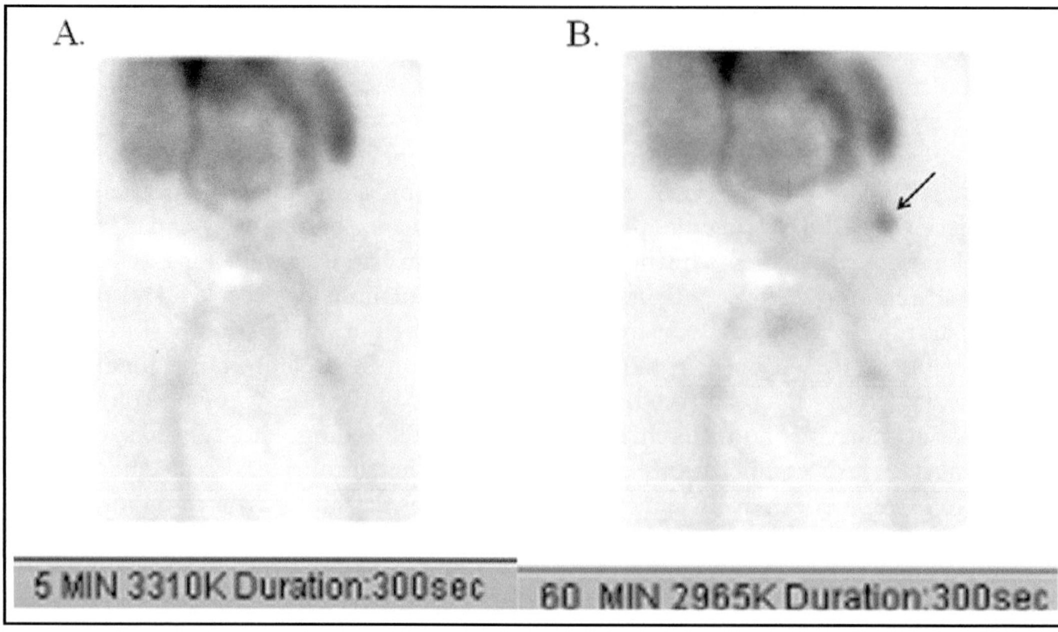

Figure 11-2. (A) Baseline tagged RBC scan. (B) Tagged RBC scan with active bleeding from the left colon.

Figure 11-3. Angiography with active bleeding from the right colon.

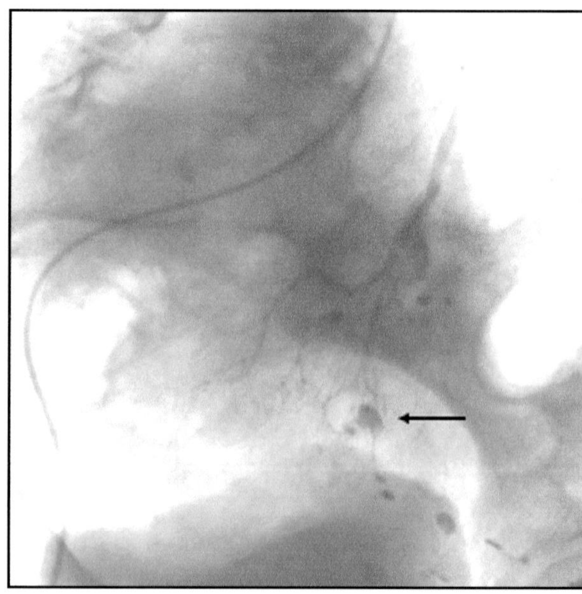

Angiography

A more rapid bleeding rate (at least 0.5 to 1.5 mL/min) is necessary for detection during angiography (Figure 11-3) compared with a tagged RBC scan. Patients who are bleeding massively and hemodynamically unstable should be resuscitated and proceed directly to angiography without a tagged RBC scan or to surgery. The diagnostic yield of angiography ranges from 27% to 77%, with a sensitivity and specificity of 47% and 100%, respectively.[8] Minor complications of angiography occur in 26% of patients, whereas major complications resulting in death or surgery can occur in as many as 17%

Table 11-1. Common Sources of Gastrointestinal Bleeding and Prevalence

SOURCE	PREVALENCE, %
Diverticulosis	17 to 44
Colonic angiodysplasia	2 to 30
Ischemia	9 to 21
Malignant neoplasm	4 to 14
Hemorrhoids/anorectal	4 to 11
Postpolypectomy	1 to 6
Unknown	8 to 12

of patients. Complications include renal failure, hematoma, ischemia, and infarction. Provocative testing using anticoagulants (eg, intravenous heparin and intra-arterial tissue plasminogen activator) to promote bleeding and vasodilators (intra-arterial tolazoline) can increase diagnostic yield, although there is a concern for significant complications, including death. Additional studies are necessary to optimize the efficacy and prove the safety of this approach.

Multidetector-Row Computed Tomography

Multidetector-row computed tomography (MDCT) can detect bleeding rates of 0.3 mL/min and incorporates several computed tomography (CT) improvements, which allow enhanced delineation of mesenteric vessels: faster scanning time, more accurate acquisition of images in arterial and venous phases, and improved 3-dimensional display. Patients do not ingest any water or contrast material orally, and after an initial unenhanced CT scan, images are obtained during the arterial phase to identify extravasation of contrast into the bowel lumen. Studies demonstrate 91% to 92% sensitivity and near 100% specificity for detecting the source of acute GI bleeding with MDCT and 100% accuracy in localization of the bleeding site.[9] Although MDCT is promising, additional studies are needed to determine the optimal role of MDCT in lower GI bleeding.

Differential Diagnosis

The differential diagnosis of acute lower GI bleeding is broad, although the vast majority of cases result from diverticulosis, ischemic colitis, angiodysplasias, neoplasia, and hemorrhoids (Table 11-1). Despite evaluation, the cause of lower GI bleeding may go undetected in approximately 12% of cases.[10,11]

Diverticulosis

Diverticulosis is the most common cause of significant lower GI bleeding. It is more prevalent in developed countries and older patients. Diverticulosis occurs in 5% to 10% of people younger than 40 years compared with more than half of people older than 80 years.

Approximately 75% to 80% of people with diverticulosis are asymptomatic, whereas 3% to 20% experience diverticular bleeding, with massive bleeding in 3% to 5% of patients. Recurrent diverticular bleeding occurs in 25% to 35% of patients, and 50% of these people experience a third episode of diverticular hemorrhage.[12]

Risk factors for diverticular bleeding include the use of NSAIDs and advanced age. Bleeding can occur anywhere in the colon. Bleeding occurs at the site of penetration of the vasa recta, with the vasa recta stretched over the dome of the diverticula, resulting in segmental wall weakness and predisposing to rupture. Abrupt painless bleeding characterizes diverticular bleeding; mild lower abdominal cramping may occur before the passage of bright red or maroon blood because of the cathartic nature of blood in the intestines. Melena is unusual in patients with diverticular bleeding.

If a bleeding diverticulum is identified during colonoscopy, there are multiple endoscopic therapeutic options, including epinephrine injection, bipolar coagulation, combination therapy, and mechanical therapy.[13] Once a bleeding diverticulum is identified, it is often helpful to mark the location of the diverticulum in question with a tattoo or via the placement of endoscopic clips if additional endoscopic, angiographic, or surgical therapy is necessary. Epinephrine injection in 4 quadrants can control bleeding or close the mouth of the diverticulum by tamponade. Most bleeding vessels or nonbleeding visible vessels identified during endoscopy are located on the neck of the diverticulum. Thermal therapy should be avoided at the dome of the diverticulum given the risk of perforation. Bipolar coagulation can be performed with 10 to 15 W of power, mild-moderate pressure, and short 1-second pulses. Clots can be removed using the cold guillotine technique (similar to the technique for upper GI bleeding), and the underlying area can be irrigated vigorously to expose any stigmata of bleeding; any underlying lesion should be treated appropriately.

Limited data from small studies suggest that endoscopic treatment is successful long term. Case series report successful treatment of bleeding diverticula using mechanical therapy with endoclips or endoscopic band ligation (Figure 11-4). The technique of hemoclip placement is to target the bleeding vessel, which is often located at the neck of the diverticulum. Although a small diverticulum may be completely closed by this technique, this zipper technique is not adequate to treat bleeding from larger diverticula because it may not target the bleeding vessel and ongoing bleeding may occur.

Angiography offers another treatment option for patients with bleeding from diverticulosis. Continuous, selective intra-arterial vasopressin infusion stops bleeding in approximately 90% of cases, with as many as 50% rebleeding after the infusion is discontinued.[14] Despite this temporary effect in many patients, vasopressin infusion can be helpful by allowing bowel preparation before a semielective definitive surgical procedure. However, it can cause abdominal pain and should be avoided in patients with known coronary artery disease.

Superselective embolization uses 2.5- to 3-Fr microcatheters, which are advanced through conventional 5-Fr catheters to access smaller, more distal vessels. Various embolic agents are used, including gel foam, polyvinyl alcohol, and microcoils. Treatment success ranges from 44% to 91%, with rebleeding rates ranging from 6% to 34%. Recurrent bleeding 1 month after embolization occurs in less than 15% of patients with diverticular hemorrhage compared with more than 40% with nondiverticular causes, such as AVM.[15]

Persistent massive hemorrhage, transfusion requirement exceeding 4 units in 24 hours, and recurrent diverticular bleeding are potential indications for surgery, which occurs in

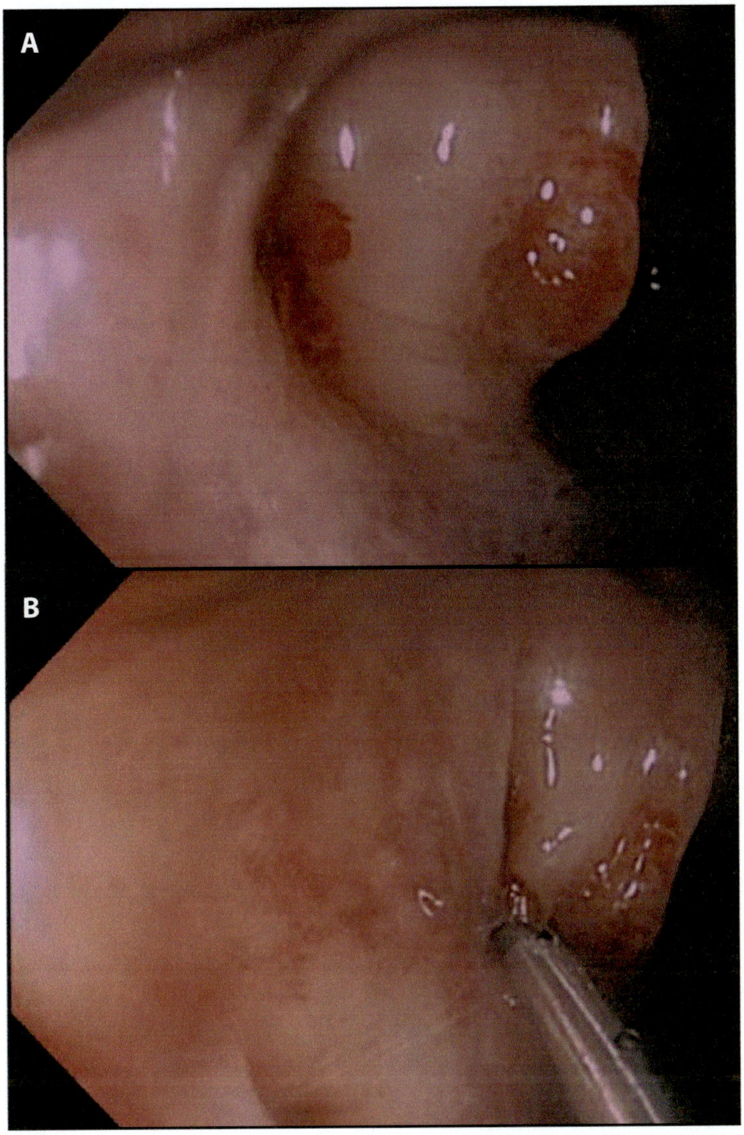

Figure 11-4. (A) Diverticulum with oozing. (B) Diverticular bleeding controlled with clips.

18% to 25% of patients requiring transfusions for diverticular bleeding. Blind segmental resection should be avoided because of high rebleeding (as high as 33%) and mortality rates (20% to 57%). Rebleeding rates as low as 0% with mortality rates ranging from 0% to 33% have been reported for blind subtotal colectomy. Mortality is lowest at 10% with directed segmental resection, with a rebleeding rate of 14% at 1-year follow-up. Therefore, efforts to localize a bleeding site before surgery should be aggressive.[16]

Angiodysplasias

Angiodysplasias are the reported source of lower GI bleeding in 3% to 40% of patients, with more than half located in the right colon. They are believed to result from degeneration of submucosal venules. Bleeding angiodysplasias are first seen with painless hematochezia similar to diverticular hemorrhage in 47% of patients or chronic, intermittent

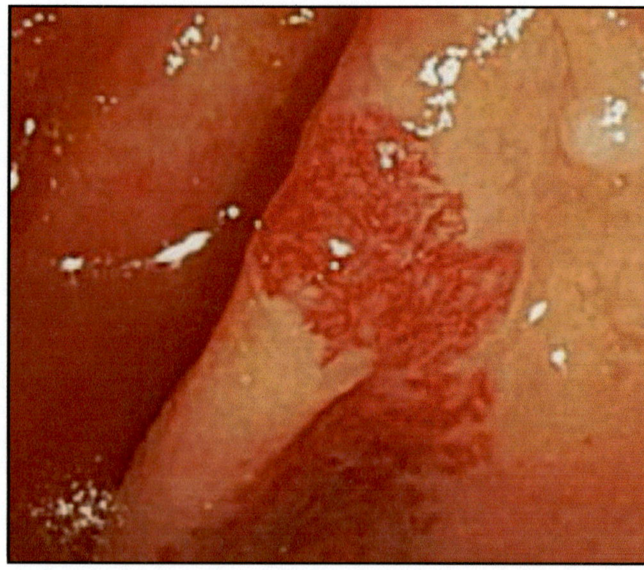

Figure 11-5. Colonic AVM.

bleeding. Risk factors for bleeding include patient age older than 60 years, right-sided location, and certain conditions, including aortic stenosis and chronic renal failure.[17]

Angiography is considered the gold standard in diagnosing angiodysplasias. Findings include ectatic, slowly emptying veins; vascular tufts; or early-filling veins. On colonoscopy, angiodysplasia has a characteristic appearance of a 2- to 10-mm, red, fernlike, flat lesion with ectatic vessels radiating from a central vessel (Figure 11-5). Poor bowel preparation and use of meperidine and other opiates, which transiently decrease mucosal blood flow, could potentially hinder the identification of angiodysplasias. The use of naloxone may improve detection of angiodysplasias during colonoscopy.

Bleeding angiodysplasias discovered during colonoscopy can be treated with a variety of thermal therapies. Electrocautery should begin with the outer feeder vessels and progress toward the central vessel. Argon plasma coagulation (APC) has become a popular noncontact method, with a reported success rate of 77% to 83%.[18] If there is a history of guaiac-positive stool or iron deficiency anemia, angiodysplasias should be treated even if not actively bleeding at the time of colonoscopy. Nonbleeding angiodysplasias without evidence of GI bleeding should not be treated.

Ischemic Colitis

The diagnosis of colonic ischemia is established by a combination of clinical setting, physical diagnosis, and diagnostic studies. The differential diagnosis includes infectious colitis, inflammatory bowel disease, diverticulitis, radiation enteritis, and colon cancer. *Clostridium difficile* infection must be excluded in patients admitted to the hospital. Although there are no specific blood tests for colonic ischemia, elevations may be observed in the white blood cell count and in amylase, creatine phosphokinase, and serum lactate levels. Most plain radiographs in patients with colonic ischemia have nonspecific findings, although thumbprinting due to submucosal edema and pneumatosis may typically be seen in patients with more advanced disease. CT scans may reveal segmental thickening of the involved colon, which in and of itself is a nonspecific finding. Although colonic ischemia commonly occurs in the watershed areas of the colon that lie between the end circulations

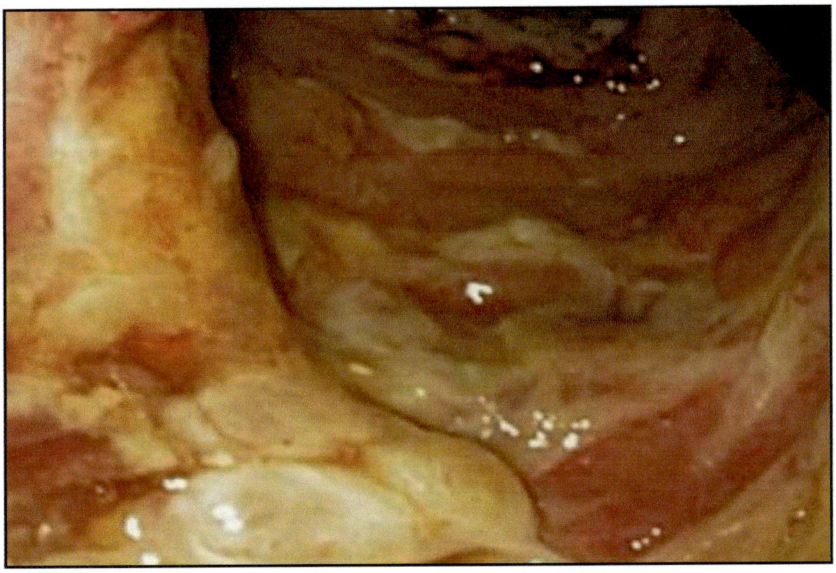

Figure 11-6. Ischemic colitis.

of arteries and typically results from low flow, it may result from a thromboembolic event in the right colon because of emboli in the ileocolic artery.

Endoscopic evaluation with sigmoidoscopy or colonoscopy is often used to confirm the diagnosis in patients whose diagnosis is unclear and who do not have signs of peritonitis or perforation. Care must be taken to avoid overdistention with air during the examination to prevent worsening ischemic damage. Endoscopic findings typically occur in a segmental distribution and vary depending on the degree of damage, ranging from pale mucosa with petechial bleeding to cyanotic, necrotic bowel (Figure 11-6). Angiography is usually not indicated because the blood flow to the colon returns to normal by the time of clinical presentation.

Neoplasm

In patients older than 50 years, a colonic neoplasm causes approximately 10% of rectal bleeding.[19] Although most bleeding from colonic neoplasms tends to be low grade and occult, bleeding may occasionally be brisk and overt. Bleeding occurs because of erosion or ulceration of the lesion. Distal lesions (left side and rectum) are more likely to manifest with bright red blood per rectum, whereas more proximal lesions tend to manifest with maroon stool, melena, or occult blood.

Colonoscopy with biopsies typically confirms the diagnosis of a neoplasm, although larger neoplasms may be detected on CT scans. The therapeutic options for patients with bleeding neoplasms are limited. Standard endoscopic therapies have marginal effectiveness. The treatment for most patients with bleeding colonic neoplasms includes radiation therapy and/or surgical resection.

Hemorrhoids

Hemorrhoids and other anorectal disorders (solitary rectal ulcers and anal fissures) are an important source of lower GI bleeding. Hemorrhoids are dilated submucosal vessels in the anus that are considered internal if above the dentate line and external if below

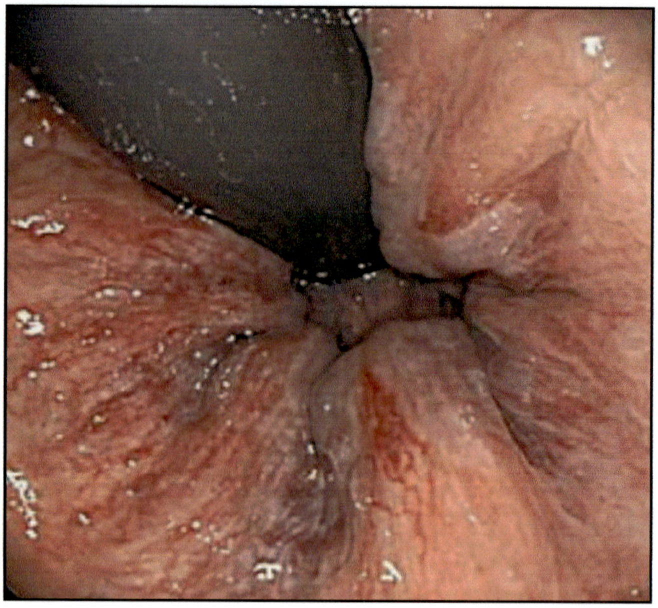

Figure 11-7. External hemorrhoids.

(Figure 11-7). They are extremely common and usually asymptomatic but can manifest with pruritus, thrombosis, or hematochezia. Bleeding from hemorrhoids occurs when a blood vessel ruptures.

The clinical manifestations of bleeding hemorrhoids include painless hematochezia with the stool coated by bright red blood and, less commonly, with blood dripping into the toilet bowl or staining underwear. Although hemorrhoidal bleeding is usually low grade, massive bleeding rarely may occur, especially in patients with coagulopathy. Acute treatment for most patients with bleeding hemorrhoids is not needed because most episodes are mild and resolve spontaneously. Topical medical treatments help decrease inflammation, and band ligation successfully treats bleeding hemorrhoids. Rarely, surgery is needed for those with persistent or massive bleeding.

Postpolypectomy Bleeding

Postpolypectomy bleeding occurs after 1% to 6% of polypectomies and is the leading major complication after colonoscopy with polypectomy.[18] Therapeutic options include resnaring the stalk of the polypectomy site to apply pressure, injection with epinephrine, contact or noncontact thermal treatment with bipolar coagulation or argon plasma coagulation, and endoclip application (Figure 11-8). Although bleeding usually occurs within 7 days, delayed bleeding can occur as long as 30 days after polypectomy when the eschar falls off the site. Polypectomy bleeding is usually self-limited, and more than 70% of cases resolve with supportive care.

Risk factors for postpolypectomy bleeding include removal of large polyps (especially larger than 2 cm in diameter), patient age older than 65 years, cardiovascular or chronic renal disease, platelet dysfunction, and coagulopathy. Multiple studies have tried to identify techniques to reduce the risk of postpolypectomy bleeding. Submucosal injection of saline has proved useful in large polyps, as well as placement of prophylactic endoclips in polyps larger than 2 cm to prevent bleeding.[20] A meta-analysis suggested that use of one injection or a combination of injections with epinephrine or saline and endoscopic clipping reduces

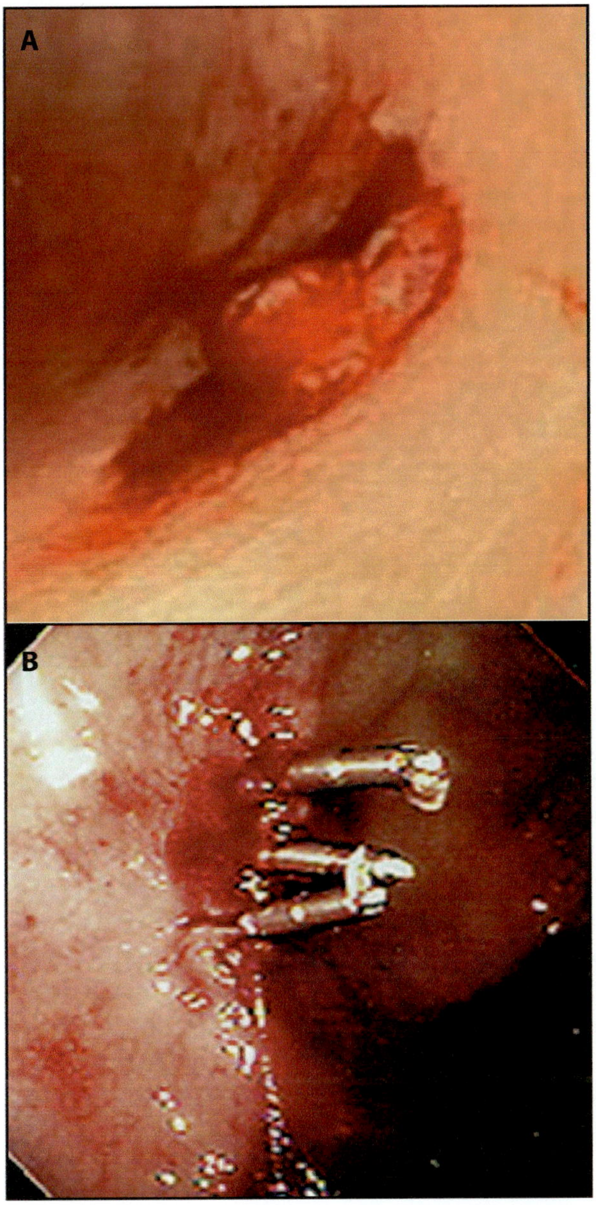

Figure 11-8. (A) Postpolypectomy bleeding. (B) Bleeding controlled with clips.

the risk of early rebleeding.[21] In patients being treated with anticoagulation or antiplatelet agents, the use of prophylactic hemoclips in polyps larger than 1 cm may reduce bleeding.

Radiation Proctitis

Pelvic radiation can cause both acute and chronic radiation proctitis. Acute damage manifests within 3 months of radiation therapy, with diarrhea, tenesmus, and, rarely, bleeding. Chronic radiation proctitis typically occurs 9 to 14 months after radiation in as many as 20% of patients but may occur years later (Figure 11-9).[22] Bleeding is a prominent symptom caused by mucosal atrophy and fibrosis, which result in chronic mucosal ischemia.

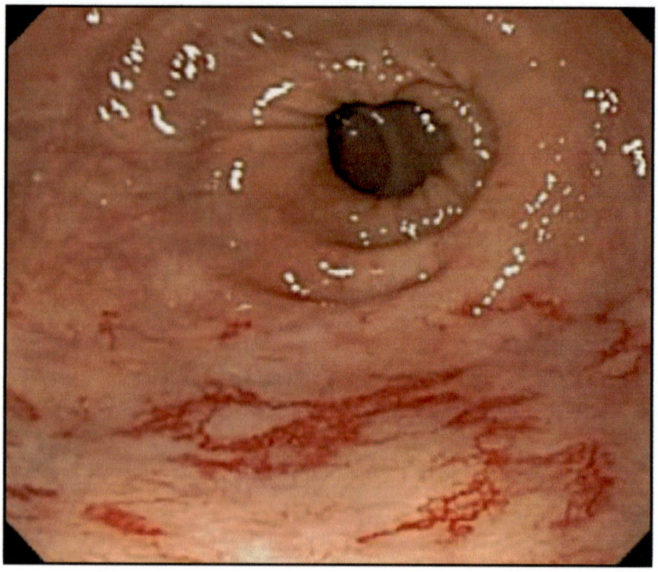

Figure 11-9. Chronic radiation proctitis.

There are no standardized recommendations for treatment of bleeding from radiation proctitis. Endoscopic therapy appears superior to medical treatment in reducing severe bleeding, with nearly 75% success after endoscopic treatment compared with 33% for medical therapy.[23] Heater probe and bipolar coagulation have proved effective in controlling bleeding during a mean of 4 treatment sessions performed every 4 to 6 weeks. APC has received more attention recently, with 85% to 100% success in reducing or stopping bleeding during a mean of 2 to 3 treatments every 4 to 8 weeks. During long-term follow-up for a period of 1 to 5 years, recurrent bleeding occurred in 0% to 8% of patients.[24] All visible telangiectasias are obliterated at each session if possible, although this may not be feasible in patients with significant disease, whereas rectal ulcers resulting from previous treatments are avoided. Short-term complications occur in 7% of patients and include rectal pain and fever. Rare major complications include rectovaginal fistula, anal or rectal stricture, and perforation. A full bowel preparation is required for APC because there have been reports of gas explosions resulting in perforations during APC with an enema preparation. A newer endoscopic ablation technique involves radiofrequency ablation, with case reports of successful treatment of radiation proctitis in patients in whom APC failed.[25]

Hyperbaric oxygen, although available in a limited manner, is another therapeutic option in patients with radiation proctitis that promotes angiogenesis and collagen formation, leading to reepithelialization. A meta-analysis suggests that hyperbaric oxygen therapy is effective in radiation proctitis.[26] The treatment regimen is rigorous, with patients placed in a hyperbaric chamber at a pressure of 2 to 2.5 atm with 100% oxygen for 90 minutes, 5 to 7 days per week for 20 to 80 sessions.[27] Hyperbaric oxygen therapy may be considered before proceeding to surgery in patients refractory to standard medical and endoscopic treatment.

REFERENCES

1. Bosch J, Thabut D, Albillos A, et al. Recombinant factor VIIa for variceal bleeding in patients with advanced cirrhosis: a randomized controlled trial. *Hepatology.* 2008;47:1604-1614.
2. Davila RE, Rajan E, Adler DG, et al. Standards of Practice Committee. ASGE Guideline: the role of endoscopy in the patient with lower GI bleeding. *Gastrointest Endosc.* 2005;62:656-660.
3. Lhewa DY, Strate LL. Pros and cons of colonoscopy in management of acute lower gastrointestinal bleeding. *World J Gastroenterol.* 2012;18:1185-1190.
4. Strate LL, Ayanian JZ, Kotler G, Syngal S. Risk factors for mortality in lower intestinal bleeding. *Clin Gastroenterol Hepatol.* 2008;6:1004-1010.
5. Velayos FS, Williamson A, Sousa KH, et al. Early predictors of severe lower gastrointestinal bleeding and adverse outcomes: a prospective study. *Clin Gastroenterol Hepatol.* 2004;2:485-490.
6. Green BT, Rockey DC, Portwood G, et al. Urgent colonoscopy for evaluation and management of acute lower gastrointestinal hemorrhage: a randomized controlled trial. *Am J Gastroenterol.* 2005;100:2395-2402.
7. Laine L, Shah A. Randomized trial of urgent vs. elective colonoscopy in patients hospitalized with lower GI bleeding. *Am J Gastroenterol.* 2010;105:2636-2641.
8. Maleux G, Roeflaer F, Heye S, et al. Long-term outcome of transcatheter embolotherapy for acute lower gastrointestinal hemorrhage. *Am J Gastroenterol.* 2009;104:2042-2046.
9. Geffroy Y, Rodallec MH, Boulay-Coletta I, Julles MC, Ridereau-Zins C, Zins M. Multidetector CT angiography in acute gastrointestinal bleeding: why, when, and how. *Radiographics.* 2011;31(3):E35-E46.
10. Longstreth G. Epidemiology and outcome of patients hospitalized with acute lower gastrointestinal hemorrhage: a population-based study. *Am J Gastroenterol.* 1997;92:419-424.
11. Strate LL, Orav EJ, Syngal S. Early predictors of severity in acute lower intestinal tract bleeding. *Arch Intern Med.* 2003;163:838-843.
12. Petruzziello L, Iacopini F, Bulajic M, et al. Review article: uncomplicated diverticular disease of the colon. *Aliment Pharmacol Ther.* 2006;23:1379-1391.
13. Song LWK, Baron TH. Endoscopic management of acute lower gastrointestinal bleeding. *Am J Gastroenterol.* 2008;103:1881-1887.
14. Darcy M. Treatment of lower gastrointestinal bleeding: vasopressin infusion versus embolization. *J Vasc Interv Radiol.* 2003;14(5):535-543.
15. Tan KK, Wong D, Sim R. Superselective embolization for lower gastrointestinal hemorrhage: an institutional review over 7 years. *World J Surg.* 2008;32:2707-2715.
16. Schuetz A, Jauch KW. Lower gastrointestinal bleeding: therapeutic strategies, surgical techniques, and results. *Langenbecks Arch Surg.* 2001;386:17-25.
17. Strate LL. Lower GI bleeding: epidemiology and diagnosis. *Gastroenterol Clin N Am.* 2005;34:643-664.
18. Kwan V, Bourke MJ, Williams SJ, et al. Argon plasma coagulation in the management of symptomatic gastrointestinal vascular lesions: experience in 100 consecutive patients with long-term follow-up. *Am J Gastroenterol.* 2006;101:58-63.
19. Hreinssona JP, Gujmundssonb S, Kalaitzakisc E, Bjornssona ES. Lower gastrointestinal bleeding: incidence, etiology, and outcomes in a population-based setting. *Eur J Gastroenterol Hepatol.* 2012;25:37-43.
20. Liaquat H, Rohn E, Rex DK. Prophylactic clip closure reduced the risk of delayed postpolypectomy hemorrhage: experience in 277 clipped large sessile or flat colorectal lesions and 247 control lesions. *Gastrointest Endosc.* 2013;77:401-407.
21. Li LY, Liu QS, Li L, et al. A meta-analysis and systematic review of prophylactic endoscopic treatments for postpolypectomy bleeding. *Int J Colorectal Dis.* 2011;26(6):709-719.
22. Hong JJ, Park W, Ehrenpreis ED. Review article: current therapeutic options for radiation proctopathy. *Aliment Pharmacol Ther.* 2001;15:1253-1262.
23. Jensen DM, Machicado GA, Cheng S, et al. A randomized prospective study of endoscopic bipolar electrocoagulation and heater probe treatment of chronic rectal bleeding from radiation telangiectasia. *Gastrointest Endosc.* 1997;45:20-25.
24. Karamanolis G, Triantafyllou K, Tsiamoulos Z, et al. Argon plasma coagulation has a long-lasting therapeutic effect in patients with chronic radiation proctitis. *Endoscopy.* 2009;41(6):529-531.
25. Eddi R, DePasquale JR. Radiofrequency ablation for the treatment of radiation proctitis: a case report and review of literature. *Therap Adv Gastroenterol.* 2013;6(1):69-76.

26. Bennett MH, Feldmeier J, Hampson N, Smee R, Milross C. Hyperbaric oxygen therapy for late radiation tissue injury. *Cochrane Database Syst Rev.* 2012 May 16;5:CD005005.
27. Clarke RE, Tenorio LMC, Hussey JR, et al. Hyperbaric oxygen treatment of chronic refractory radiation proctitis: a randomized and controlled double-blind crossover trial with long-term follow-up. *Int J Radiat Oncol Biol Phys.* 2008;72:134-143.

Please visit www.routledge.com/9781617116148 to access additional material.

12

Colonoscopy Quality Indicators in Training and Beyond
What You Need to Know

Jonathan Cohen, MD, FASGE, FACG

The goal of colonoscopy training is to provide future endoscopists with the technical and cognitive skills required to independently perform a high-quality procedure. What does the term *high-quality* mean in the context of colonoscopy? To know the goals of training, to know how to objectively assess the competency of trainees, and to gauge actual procedure performance in subsequent practice, we need to have a consensus about the specific parameters that constitute a high-quality examination. To set the bar for these parameters, it is necessary to have benchmarking data pertaining to performance of the procedure in the community. However, to determine what to measure, we must begin with a common understanding and agreement about what really matters concerning the procedure.

To this end, the American Society for Gastrointestinal Endoscopy/American College of Gastroenterology Taskforce on Quality in Endoscopy was created in 2005 and published a set of 5 documents in 2006. In these papers, the Taskforce defined a set of quality indicators common to all endoscopic procedures and specific to esophagogastroduodenoscopy (EGD), colonoscopy, endoscopic retrograde cholangiopancreatoscopy (ERCP), and endoscopic ultrasound (EUS).

Quality Indicators

The indicators for colonoscopy include those common to all endoscopic procedures (Table 12-1)[1] and those particular to colonoscopy (Table 12-2).[2] The list is composed of practices that have been linked to good patient outcomes, items for which there would likely be disparities in practice among providers, and items amenable to measurement.

Adler DG, ed.
Core Concepts in Colonoscopy (pp 159-164).

Table 12-1. Summary of Proposed Quality Indicators for Endoscopic Procedures

QUALITY INDICATOR	GRADE OF RECOMMENDATION[a]
1. Proper indication	1C+
2. Informed consent	3
3. History and physical examination	3
4. Risk stratification	1C
5. Prophylactic antibiotics	2C
6. Timeliness recorded	3
7. Sedation plan recorded	3
8. Anticoagulants recorded	3
9. Team pause	3
10. Photodocumentation of major abnormalities	3
11. Patient monitoring	3
12. Medications documented	3
13. Reversal agents	3
14. Discharge criteria	3
15. Discharge instructions	3
16. Pathology follow-up	3
17. Procedure report	3
18. Reporting of complications	3
19. Patient satisfaction	3
20. Communication with referring provider(s)	3
21. Plan for postprocedure resumption of anticoagulants	3

[a]Refer to Table 12-3 for an explanation of Grades of Recommendation.

This table of potential quality indicators was meant to be a comprehensive listing of measurable endpoints. It is not the intention of the Taskforce that all endpoints be measured in every practice setting. In most cases, validation may be required before a given endpoint may be adopted universally.

Each quality indicator is classified as either a process or outcome measure. Process measures indicate the presence or absence of an action that is presumed to be a surrogate or predictor of a clinically relevant outcome. Outcome measures are metrics that measure a clinically relevant patient event, such as death, recurrent bleeding, or admission to a hospital. The relative value of a process hinges on the available evidence that supports its connection to a clinically relevant outcome. Although outcome quality indicators are preferred, many

Table 12-2. Summary of Proposed Quality Indicators for Colonoscopy

QUALITY INDICATOR	GRADE OF RECOMMENDATION[a]
1. Appropriate indication	1C+
2. Informed consent obtained, including specific discussion of risks associated with colonoscopy	3
3. Use of recommended postpolypectomy and postcancer-resection surveillance intervals	1A
4. Use of recommended ulcerative colitis/Crohn's surveillance intervals	2C
5. Documentation of the quality of the preparation in the procedure note	2C
6. Cecal intubation rates (visualization of the cecum by notation of landmarks and photodocumentation of landmarks should be performed in every procedure)	1C
7. Detection of adenomas in asymptomatic individuals (screening)	1C
8. Withdrawal time: mean withdrawal time should be more than 6 min in normal colonoscopies performed in patients with intact anatomy	2C
9. Biopsy specimens obtained from patients with chronic diarrhea	2C
10. Number and distribution of biopsy samples in ulcerative colitis and Crohn's colitis surveillance. Goal: 4 per 10-cm section of involved colon or approximately 32 biopsy specimens per case of pancolitis	1C
11. Mucosally based pedunculated polyps and sessile polyps less than 2 cm in size should be resected endoscopically or unresectability documented	3
12. Complication rates: incidence of perforation by procedure type (all indications vs screening) and postpolypectomy bleeding	2C
13. Postpolypectomy bleeding managed nonoperatively	1C

[a]Refer to Table 12-3 for an explanation of Grades of Recommendation.

This table of potential quality indicators was meant to be a comprehensive listing of measurable endpoints. It is not the intention of the Taskforce that all endpoints be measured in every practice setting. In most cases, validation may be required before a given endpoint may be adopted universally.

Table 12-3. Grades of Recommendation

GRADE OF RECOMMENDATION	CLARITY OF BENEFIT	METHODOLOGIC STRENGTH SUPPORTING EVIDENCE	IMPLICATIONS
1A	Clear	Randomized trials without important limitations	Strong recommendation; can be applied to most clinical settings
1B	Clear	Randomized trials with important limitations (inconsistent results, nonfatal methodolgic flaws)	Strong recommendation; likely to apply to most practice settings
1C+	Clear	Overwhelming evidence from observational studies	Strong recommendation; can apply to most practice settings in most situations
1C	Clear	Observational studies	Intermediate-strength recommendation; may change when stronger evidence is available
2A	Unclear	Randomized trials without important limitations	Intermediate-strength recommendation; best action may differ depending on circumstances or patients' or societal values
2B	Unclear	Randomized trials with important limitations (inconsistent results, nonfatal methodologic flaws)	Weak recommendation; alternative approaches may be better under some circumstances
2C	Unclear	Observational studies	Very weak recommendation; alter-native approaches likely to be better under some circumstances
3	Unclear	Expert opinion only	Weak recommendation; likely to change as data become available

Adapted from Guyatt G, Sinclair J, Cook D, Jaeschke R, Schunemann H, Pauker S. Moving from evidence to action. Grading recommendations: a qualitative approach. In: Guyatt G, Rennie D, eds. *Users' Guides to the Medical Literature*. Chicago, IL: AMA Press; 2002:599-608.

are difficult to measure or are uncommon occurrences, such that they are unwieldy for routine measurement in clinical practice. In such cases, it is reasonable to use process indicators as surrogate measures of high-quality endoscopy. Quality indicators often are expressed in terms that provide direction to facilitate measurement; when possible, the wording implies a numerator of correct performance and a denominator of opportunities for correct performance for each parameter under consideration. For example, rather than "appropriate indication," the corresponding quality indicator for this parameter would be "frequency with which endoscopy is performed for a proper indication."

For each of the quality indicators, the Taskforce selected performance targets from benchmarking data in the literature when possible. It is important to emphasize that the performance targets listed do not necessarily reflect the standard of care but rather serve as specific goals to direct quality improvement efforts.

When this textbook was published, these documents were being updated to reflect the growing importance of outcome measures over process measures and a body of benchmarking data generated since 2006 that has guided our understanding of goals for performance of a number of these quality indicators.

Quality Indicators for Colonoscopy

For colonoscopy, priority indicators are (1) the adenoma detection rate (ADR), (2) the use of recommended intervals between colonoscopies performed for average-risk colorectal screening and colon polyp surveillance, and (3) the cecal intubation rate with photographic documentation.

For each of these indicators, reaching the recommended performance target is considered to be strongly associated with important clinical outcomes. These indicators can be readily measured in a manageable number of examinations, and for each there is evidence of substantial variation in performance. In addition, there is evidence for both the ADR and the use of recommended screening and surveillance intervals that simple educational and corrective measures can improve performance.[3-6]

The primary purpose of measuring quality indicators is to improve patient care by identifying poor performers and retraining them or, less commonly, removing privileges to perform colonoscopy if performance cannot be improved. For practicing colonoscopists, the ultimate justification for measuring outcomes relating to quality indicators is evidence that improving these parameters leads to a reduction in the risk of interval colorectal cancer. Demands on the part of accrediting bodies and eventually payers and patients also will serve as compelling drivers for endoscopists to routinely track their performance. Government reporting and pay-for-performance programs such as the Physician Quality Reporting System and maintenance-of-certification quality-improvement modules provide additional motivation for gastroenterologists to track quality indicators. Electronic medical record systems and the development of national registries have made it much easier to do so.

Quality Colonoscopy and Endoscopic Training

How does this relate to trainees who are soon to become practicing clinicians? First, because measuring personal performance of quality indicators will be part of their routine practice when they complete training, it makes perfect sense that trainees learn what these indicators are and get in the habit of tracking their performance along these lines throughout their training process. Beyond this, incorporating the measurement of quality indicators during training has several clear benefits.

In any field, feedback is an integral component to successful training and skill development. Measuring performance according to quality indicators emphasizes to trainees aspects of colonoscopy that are deemed most important and provides them with objective "red flags" pertaining to those parameters that need increased attention. Recording progress according to quality indicators helps ensure that trainees reach objective levels of competency by the time they complete their training period. It also fully prepares them to continue the practice of tracking their actual performance as they enter the workforce.

For all of these reasons, fellows (and practicing clinicians after training) should track some of the key colonoscopy quality indicators listed in Tables 12-1 and 12-2, such as cecal intubation rate and ADR, along with their case volumes and complication rates. Trainee performance data should be reviewed periodically to ensure that trainees are making good progress compared with their own prior work and to compare their performance with that of other fellows in the program or, if available, with benchmarking data pertaining to trainee performance at a similar stage in the learning process. Personal report cards based on colonoscopy quality-indicator data will document that a trainee is indeed ready to perform high-quality colonoscopy without supervision and eliminate the reliance on subjective assessments for subsequent credentialing.

Conclusion

Current and future endoscopists can anticipate functioning in a world where they are expected to provide high-quality colonoscopy examinations. Specific quality indicators for colonoscopy exist, and trainees (and practicing clinicians) should be aware of the key indicators and track some of their personal outcomes to ensure they are reaching their endoscopic goals on a consistent basis.

References

1. Faigel DO, Pike IM, Baron TH, et al. Quality indicators for gastrointestinal endoscopic procedures: an introduction. *Gastrointest Endosc.* 2006;63(suppl 4):S3-S9.
2. Rex DK, Petrini JL, Baron TH, et al. Quality indicators for colonoscopy. *Gastrointest Endosc.* 2006;63:S16-S28.
3. Rex DK, Bond JH, Winawer S, et al. Quality in the technical performance of colonoscopy and the continuous quality improvement process for colonoscopy: recommendations of the U.S. Multi-Society Task Force on Colorectal Cancer. *Am J Gastroenterol.* 2002;97:1296-1308.
4. Levin B, Lieberman DA, McFarland B, et al. Screening and surveillance for the early detection of colorectal cancer and adenomatous polyps, 2008: a joint guideline from the American Cancer Society, the US Multi-Society Task Force on Colorectal Cancer, and the American College of Radiology. *Gastroenterology.* 2008;134:1570-1595.
5. Lieberman D. A call to action—measuring the quality of colonoscopy. *N Engl J Med.* 2006;355:2588-2589.
6. Kaminski MF, Regula J, Kraszewska E, et al. Quality indicators for colonoscopy and the risk of interval cancer. *N Engl J Med.* 2010;362:1795-1803.

Financial Disclosures

Dr. Douglas G. Adler is a consultant to Boston Scientific.

Dr. Todd H. Baron has received an honorarium from Boston Scientific and research support from Cook Medical and is a consultant to W.L. Gore & Associates, Inc, Pinnacle Biologics, and Cumberland Pharmaceuticals, Inc.

Dr. Kathryn R. Byrne has no financial or proprietary interest in the materials presented herein.

Dr. Jonathan Cohen has no financial or proprietary interest in the materials presented herein.

Dr. Serag Dredar has no financial or proprietary interest in the materials presented herein.

Dr. Tolga Erim has no financial or proprietary interest in the materials presented herein.

Dr. Norio Fukami has no financial or proprietary interest in the materials presented herein.

Dr. Vivek Kaul has no financial or proprietary interest in the materials presented herein.

Dr. Gyanprakash Ketwaroo has no financial or proprietary interest in the materials presented herein.

Dr. C. Andrew Kistler has no financial or proprietary interest in the materials presented herein.

Dr. Shivangi Kothari has no financial or proprietary interest in the materials presented herein.

Dr. Linda S. Lee has no financial or proprietary interest in the materials presented herein.

Dr. John G. Lieb II has no financial or proprietary interest in the materials presented herein.

Dr. Douglas Pleskow is a consultant to and serves on the Biliary Medical Advisory Board for Boston Scientific and is a consultant to and serves on the Medical Advisory Board for Beacon Endoscopic.

Dr. Waqar Qureshi has no financial or proprietary interest in the materials presented herein.

Dr. John R. Saltzman has no financial or proprietary interest in the materials presented herein.

Dr. Robert E. Sedlack has no financial or proprietary interest in the materials presented herein.

Dr. Ali Siddiqui has no financial or proprietary interest in the materials presented herein.

Dr. Anna Strongin has no financial or proprietary interest in the materials presented herein.

Dr. Shou-Jiang Tang has no financial or proprietary interest in the materials presented herein.

Dr. Jeffrey L. Tokar is a consultant to Boston Scientific and has received support (in the form of honoraria and travel/lodging expenses) for conference presentations and faculty participation from Olympus Medical, Fujifilm, and Novartis, and for membership on a data safety monitoring board for Augmenix, Inc. Dr. Tokar has no financial or proprietary interest in the materials presented herein.

Dr. Melissa A. Verrengia has no financial or proprietary interest in the materials presented herein.

Dr. Nicolas Villa has no financial or proprietary interest in the materials presented herein.

Dr. Louis M. Wong Kee Song has no financial or proprietary interest in the materials presented herein.

For Product Safety Concerns and Information please contact our
EU representative GPSR@taylorandfrancis.com Taylor & Francis
Verlag GmbH, Kaufingerstraße 24, 80331 München, Germany